THE CANDIDA SYNDROME

By Kay Hitchen

First published in 2000 by **KennedySmith (Press) Ltd**
ISBN 1-903379-00-8

Copyright © 2000 Kay Hitchen

This book was designed and produced by:

KennedySmith (Press) Ltd,
21 Whittle Place,
South Newmoor,
Irvine KA11 4HP.

The information in this book is not intended to replace the advice of
your medical practitioner. The author and publishers are not
responsible for any adverse consequences resulting from the use
or misuse of the information in this book.

THE CANDIDA SYNDROME

EVERYBODY'S DIFFERENT in the fight against Candida. This is a 'Do–it–yourself' method of finding the best treatment for each individual. It includes diet sheets and recipes to help you navigate your way around 'the fungal jungle'.

By Kay Hitchen

A NOTE TO THE READER

The information contained in this book is generalised and should not be regarded as specific for any individual patient. If you are in any doubt about your health you should consult a competent doctor or complementary health practitioner.

The author and the publisher cannot accept legal responsibility for any problem arising out of experimentation with the methods described in this book.

THE CANDIDA SYNDROME

Contents

FOREWORD
by
Jan de Vries

Some time ago I had a very interesting conversation with an eminent Doctor from Glasgow. We were discussing the importance of the immune system and how this is now being attacked by our diet, the air we breathe, stress and our life style. This Doctor questioned the possibility that ME could come out of an imbalance in our diet, and also as a result of stress, and his views were certainly typical of how Doctors then felt about ME.

Thankfully, times have changed and now most of the Doctors and General Practitioners will agree that ME or the Post Viral Syndrome exists, and certainly there has been a lot of research done by the orthodox medical profession regarding this. However there is another result of a weak immune system, which has yet to be recognised by the medical profession – this is a chronic Candida problem. From my experience a chronic Candida problem can mimic a lot of many different illnesses and sometimes the diagnosis can be difficult. The orthodox medical profession has yet to see that this is possible, and most Doctors still do not accept that such a condition can exist.

Kay Hitchen is a practitioner who has a vast amount of experience with Candida and how it can wreak havoc in the lives of many. The diagnosis of Candida and how it can be helped is a very complex issue and this book will be very useful for those who have been confused by the many symptoms that can arise and more importantly how to handle and manage these symptoms. Kay is in the forefront of research into the treatment of Candida problems, and I feel that many will benefit from her experience and insight into this sometimes very difficult problem.

It is only with this continuing educational process that we can learn more about Candida and how it can affect our health, and also more importantly to get others and particularly the orthodox medical profession to accept that it can be a cause of serious illness. As Doctors now have accepted that ME exists, I have no doubt that with books like this we will, before too long, be able to understand more about Candida.

WHAT IS CANDIDA?

Over 80% of women, and many men and children suffer from Candida and yet it is a condition that is still not recognised by many medical doctors.

Candida is a yeast fungus that lives in the large intestine. We all have it, and to a certain extent, the yeast can be helpful for our digestion. However, if there is an overgrowth of the organism, a multitude of problems can arise. Quite often the symptoms appear relatively minor, but constantly suffering from many minor symptoms can make life into one major problem.

Patients often ask, "How does the yeast get out of control?" The reasons for this are obviously quite complex. If the body's immune system has been weakened, the yeast organisms will multiply and grow uncontrollably.

Our immune system can be regarded as the 'policemen' that we have inside us. In our blood stream (and throughout our body), there are white blood cells or lymphocytes, which are the policemen 'on the beat'. These cells are responsible for recognising what is right or wrong, and if there is something to correct, it is the white blood cells that do the work.

For example, the white cells in the body recognise the presence of viruses that would cause a cold, and they mount a challenge and attack these invading organisms.

When the 'policemen' in our body are weakened, more crime takes place, and therefore we are subject to more infections. Some of these infections can become chronic, leading to post-viral fatigue or ME, and also chronic Candidiasis problems. It is interesting that a defective immune system is also responsible for the production of allergies. Some of the more troublesome symptoms of a Candida problem can be due to allergies.

Treatment of the condition can be almost as varied as the symptoms. Even natural medicine practitioners differ in their approach. However, one thing on which they are all agreed is that diet is vitally important. Candida thrives on yeast and sugar based food, and will often 'con' the body into craving the things it needs to survive. Therefore, you should avoid all forms of sugar, yeast and fungus.

THERE IS NO OVERNIGHT CURE. Treatment is often slow and frustrating; you may feel you are taking three steps forward and one step back. It is not an easy condition to treat and requires considerable willpower to stick rigidly to the initially very restricted diet. Don't be downhearted! It will be worth it in the end.

There are many excellent books available on the subject of Candida, but the list of recommended supplements in them seems to go on for ever. But what are the supplements for? Are you getting enough of the things you need? Are you taking too much of the things that are not really necessary? Are you taking the things that are right <u>for you</u>?

The information contained in any book is no substitute for a one-to-one consultation with a qualified practitioner. However, if you answer the questionnaires *(see page 7)* and heed the advice, you should obtain considerable relief from your symptoms.

WHAT IS PHYTOTHERAPY?

Apart from the correct diet and the right amount of vitamins and minerals, most of the remedies I use are Phytotherapeutic tinctures, which may be new to some people.

Phytotherapy is the use of medicinal herbs in the treatment and prevention of illness. The term was first introduced into French literature about 150 years ago, and is now widely used on the continent.

It is the forerunner of modern medicine, as we know it in the West. Evidence of the use of herbs in treating various illnesses can be traced right back in history. In the Bible there are many references to herbs being used for food and medicine. The use of herbs as medicines has also been mentioned for centuries in the literature of past cultures such as the Greeks, Egyptians and Chinese.

Medical herbalists have been using alcoholic tinctures for over 150 years. They consider it one of the best methods of extracting and preserving a medicinal herb. A tincture with an alcohol concentration of 40% to 60% has the advantage of achieving a good balance of the water soluble and fat-soluble constituents of each plant. This balance is important in reflecting the proportions of each constituent of the plant, in its fresh and original state.

Another major advantage of herbal tinctures is that the alcohol acts as a natural preservative. It avoids problems of deterioration in the quality of the herb during storage, either due to 'ageing', or bacterial and fungal contamination. The composition of the plant material can change when heat is used to create dried herbs and the more delicate constituent parts are often destroyed. With phytotherapy this does not occur.

The absorption of alcoholic tinctures is also very much better than with herb tablets. It is well known that some tablets can pass straight through the body without being absorbed at all. Tinctures, on the other hand, are assimilated through the mouth and throat, as well as through the lining of the stomach.

Absorption of a medicine through the mouth and throat has the advantage of bypassing the liver, delivering the active components to the body tissues first.

Usually the amount of alcohol in each dose of tincture is extremely small. It does not really have to be accounted for in those who may have a dietary restriction regarding alcohol, for example, those with liver disease when taken as recommended.

Many consider that alcohol should be banned totally when treating Candida. This, in my experience, is not so. True, *alcoholic drinks* should be taken very sparingly, but this does not seem to apply to pure alcohol such as that used in medicines. If one stops for a moment to think about this, the reason becomes quite clear.

Chemicals to promote the growth of the yeast organisms are introduced to enhance the fermentation process during the manufacture of alcoholic drinks such as beers and wine. These chemicals are the things that may do the damage in those suffering from Candida. When the drinks are bottled and sold the chemicals remain, unlike pure alcohol.

Pure alcohol is obtained by distillation, which is the process used in the herbal tinctures, also for the venerated drink 'Scotch' whisky. With distillation these growth promoters are left behind, and pure alcohol is obtained. This pure alcohol does not seem to have any effect in promoting the growth of Candida in the body, for those suffering from the illness.

HOW TO TREAT CANDIDA BY GROUPS

An author can only generalise in any book (even this one), and supplements that are right for one person will not necessarily be needed by another. Having Candida can be a very expensive business – but only if you let it.

Symptoms of a Candida overgrowth are many: thrush, cystitis, depression, P.M.T., headaches, sore throats, bowel problems, fatigue – the list is endless. None of the symptoms seem major, but put them together and you have a general picture of being never well. Most patients suffer from several symptoms, but very few suffer from all of them.

Now, for the first time, you can work out your very own guide to treatment. While this may not cure all your ailments in one go it should put you well on the road to recovery for the minimum cost. The reason it may not cure all your ills is that, sadly, it is still a book and still has to generalise to a degree. However, I have tried to make it as specific as possible.

To start with, simply answer all of the following questionnaires. Mark your score to each question on every list, from A-K. Score one if the problem is occasional, two if it occurs frequently, or three if it is continual. You will find that you are answering most of the questions more than once. Don't worry – this method of treatment involves grouping symptoms to give the minimum number of products to alleviate the maximum number of problems.

Add up your scores and whichever group has the highest number is the group you fit into.

Then check your group letter in the section headed 'WHAT TO TAKE – – AND WHY' *(see page 13)*. There you will find the products listed that you need to take, along with the symptoms each remedy should alleviate in your group. In the event of having the same high score in more than one group, follow the advice for the group containing the highest number of your most severe symptoms in its list of questions.

Next, check the section headed 'ADDITIONAL ADVICE' *(see page 114)* for specific dietary or environmental tips for individual symptoms.

Remember – as your condition changes, your treatment requirements will also change. You should retest yourself by answering the same questions again in one month's time. If you find a significant change in your answers, your group will change. Then it is time for you to finish the treatment you are currently taking and start on the products advised by your new group.

GROUP A

Answer every question and mark your score as follows:

1 if the problem is occasional • **2** if it occurs frequently • **3** if it is continual

DO YOU SUFFER WITH ANY OF THE FOLLOWING SYMPTOMS?

1. Allergies?
2. Dry, watery or bleary eyes?
3. Eczema?
4. Cystitis?
5. P.M.T.?
6. Breast tenderness?
7. Frequent colds or flu?
8. Constipation?
9. Poor circulation?
10. Trouble sleeping?
11. Frequent sore throats?

Now add up your score, then answer all the questions in Group B

GROUP B

Answer every question and mark your score as follows:

1 if the problem is occasional • **2** if it occurs frequently • **3** if it is continual

DO YOU SUFFER WITH ANY OF THE FOLLOWING SYMPTOMS?

1. Eczema?
2. Catarrh?
3. Cystitis?
4. Headaches?
5. Vaginal thrush?
6. Frequent colds or flu?
7. Mouth ulcers?
8. Fatigue?
9. Lack of concentration?
10. Stress?
11. Frequent sore throats?

Now add up your score, then answer all the questions in Group C

GROUP C

Answer every question and mark your score as follows:

1 if the problem is occasional • **2** if it occurs frequently • **3** if it is continual

DO YOU SUFFER WITH ANY OF THE FOLLOWING SYMPTOMS?

1. Dry, Watery or Bleary eyes?
2. Dandruff?
3. Depression?
4. Headaches?
5. White spots, brittle or flaking nails?
6. Oral thrush?
7. Mouth ulcers?
8. Poor circulation?
9. Poor memory?
10. Lack of concentration?
11. Frequent sore throats?

Now add up your score, then answer all the questions in Group D

GROUP D

Answer every question and mark your score as follows:

1 if the problem is occasional • **2** if it occurs frequently • **3** if it is continual

DO YOU SUFFER WITH ANY OF THE FOLLOWING SYMPTOMS?

1. Allergies?
2. Dry, watery or bleary eyes?
3. Eczema?
4. P.M.T.?
5. Headaches?
6. Vaginal thrush?
7. Oral thrush?
8. Diarrhoea?
9. Poor circulation?
10. Muscle pain?
11. Wind or flatulence?

Now add up your score, then answer all the questions in Group E

GROUP E

Answer every question and mark your score as follows:

1 if the problem is occasional • **2** if it occurs frequently • **3** if it is continual

DO YOU SUFFER WITH ANY OF THE FOLLOWING SYMPTOMS?

1. Eczema?
2. Psoriasis?
3. Catarrh?
4. Headaches?
5. Frequent colds or flu?
6. Diarrhoea?
7. Fatigue?
8. Muscle pain?
9. Lack of concentration?
10. Stress?
11. Trouble sleeping?

Now add up your score, then answer all the questions in Group F

GROUP F

Answer every question and mark your score as follows:

1 if the problem is occasional • **2** if it occurs frequently • **3** if it is continual

DO YOU SUFFER WITH ANY OF THE FOLLOWING SYMPTOMS?

1. Eczema?
2. Psoriasis?
3. Catarrh?
4. Cystitis?
5. Dandruff?
6. P.M.T?
7. Breast tenderness?
8. White spots, brittle or flaking nails?
9. Constipation?
10. Muscle pain?
11. Frequent sore throats?

Now add up your score, then answer all the questions in Group G

GROUP G

Answer every question and mark your score as follows:

1 if the problem is occasional • **2** if it occurs frequently • **3** if it is continual

DO YOU SUFFER WITH ANY OF THE FOLLOWING SYMPTOMS?

1. Allergies?
2. Dandruff?
3. Depression?
4. P.M.T?
5. Breast tenderness?
6. Headaches?
7. Constipation?
8. Wind or flatulence?
9. Poor memory?
10. Lack of concentration?
11. Trouble sleeping?

Now add up your score, then answer all the questions in Group H

GROUP H

Answer every question and mark your score as follows:

1 if the problem is occasional • **2** if it occurs frequently • **3** if it is continual

DO YOU SUFFER WITH ANY OF THE FOLLOWING SYMPTOMS?

1. Allergies?
2. Dry, Watery or Bleary eyes?
3. Depression?
4. P.M.T?
5. Vaginal thrush?
6. Oral thrush?
7. Frequent colds or flu?
8. Constipation?
9. Fatigue?
10. Muscle pain?
11. Frequent sore throats?

Now add up your score, then answer all the questions in Group J

GROUP J

Answer every question and mark your score as follows:

1 if the problem is occasional • **2** if it occurs frequently • **3** if it is continual

DO YOU SUFFER WITH ANY OF THE FOLLOWING SYMPTOMS?

1. Cystitis?
2. White spots, brittle or flaking nails?
3. Oral thrush?
4. Frequent colds or flu?
5. Mouth ulcers?
6. Diarrhoea?
7. Fatigue?
8. Lack of concentration?
9. Stress?
10. Trouble sleeping?
11. Frequent sore throats?

Now add up your score, then answer all the questions in Group K

GROUP K

Answer every question and mark your score as follows:

1 if the problem is occasional • **2** if it occurs frequently • **3** if it is continual

DO YOU SUFFER WITH ANY OF THE FOLLOWING SYMPTOMS?

1. Dry, watery or bleary eyes?
2. Eczema?
3. Psoriasis?
4. Depression?
5. Headaches?
6. Fatigue?
7. Poor circulation?
8. Wind or flatulence?
9. Poor memory?
10. Lack of concentration?
11. Stress?

Now add up your score for Group K and compare it with the scores you have given to the other groups. The group with the highest score is the group you fit into.

Remember: if you have more than one group with the same highest score, follow the advice for the group that has the highest number of your most severe symptoms in its list of questions.

To find the treatment most suitable for your group turn to the next section headed 'WHAT TO TAKE AND WHY'

WHAT TO TAKE AND WHY

This book should enable most people to find the diet, and the remedies, that are suitable for them personally. In this section you will find the recommended treatments for each group. There are only three items suggested for each group because any more than this can 'confuse the system'. It is always preferable to obtain vitamins and minerals from your food – see the section headed 'DIETARY GUIDELINES'.

Some people may feel happier if they are taking extra vitamins and minerals in capsule or tablet form and advice on this is given under each group. At first glance, the list may seem rather daunting, but don't be alarmed. Most of these supplements can be found in a good multivitamin/mineral supplement. Providing you eat a good healthy and varied diet, as suggested, you should absorb all the necessary nutrients from your food.

However, if you take additional supplements, proceed with caution when you go to buy them. Always buy products from a reputable manufacturer and make sure they are clearly marked 'HYPO ALLERGENIC' and 'YEAST AND SUGAR FREE'. Ensure that sugar is not present in any of its concealed forms such as those listed in the sections headed 'DIET & RECIPES' *(see page 38)*.

WHAT TO TAKE AND WHY
GROUP A

If your highest score has occurred in Group A, you should find relief by taking the following three items:

ECHINACEA TINCTURE

This is a 'natural antibiotic' which is considered to be the prime herbal remedy for the immune system. In group A patients it has proved extremely beneficial in cases of allergies, cystitis, eczema, eye problems, frequent colds/flu, and sore throats. Take 15 drops, 3 times daily, in a little water about half an hour before meals. People suffering from HIV or Leukaemia should consult a Healthcare Professional before using this product.

KELP TABLETS

This is a natural, pure Pacific ocean algae (kelp) derivative in tablet form as a natural supplement to help your thyroid. It should also help allergies, breast tenderness and constipation. Take one tablet morning and noon before meals *DO NOT TAKE AFTER TEATIME*. This product should not be taken by anyone with high blood pressure, kidney disorders or thyroid conditions, unless under medical supervision. You should not take Kelpasan if you are taking Thyroxine or if you are allergic to iodine.

GINKGO BILOBA

Ginkgo Biloba has been used for years in China for improving the memory, where it is known as the 'memory tree'. It has been shown to improve the cerebral circulation and is useful for the prevention of strokes and transient ischaemic attacks. It can also benefit breast tenderness, circulation and eye problems. Take 15 drops in half a glass of water, three times daily before meals.

If you choose to, you could also take the following in supplementation:

BETA-CAROTENE – 2,500 IU daily should help reduce allergies, frequent colds/flu, cystitis, eczema, eye problems and sore throats.

VITAMIN B2 – 100mg daily has proved beneficial in treating eczema.

VITAMIN B3 – 100mg daily can help improve sleeping problems

VITAMIN B6 – 100mg twice daily is very useful if you are suffering from breast tenderness or sleeping problems.

BIOFLAVONOIDS – 100mg twice daily taken with Vitamin C will often reduce allergies and increase your resistance to colds and flu.

VITAMIN C – 500mg twice daily. Everybody's essential vitamin, especially helpful for allergies, breast tenderness, frequent colds/flu, constipation, cystitis, eczema, eye problems and sore throats.

CALCIUM – 1,000 mg daily can help to reduce allergies and improve relaxation and sleeping.

VITAMIN E – 400 IU daily – often called 'the circulation vitamin' it should also help reduce the frequency of colds/flu, cystitis and eczema.

EVENING PRIMROSE OIL – 500mg daily to be taken with care if you have ever had epilepsy. It can help reduce allergies, breast tenderness, circulation and eczema.

GARLIC – 300mg daily taken as a supplement and used in cooking to reduce frequent colds/flu.

FOLIC ACID – 100-200 micrograms daily should help you to sleep.

MAGNESIUM – 100-300mg daily can help reduce breast tenderness, constipation and sleeping problems.

ZINC – 10-15mg twice daily. One of the most important minerals, it can help breast tenderness, frequent colds/flu, eczema and sore throats.

WHAT TO TAKE AND WHY
GROUP B

If your highest score has occurred in Group B, you should find relief by taking the following three items:

ECHINACEA TINCTURE

This is a 'natural antibiotic' which is considered to be the prime herbal remedy for the immune system. In Group B patients it has proved extremely beneficial in cases of catarrh, cystitis, eczema, fatigue, frequent colds/flu, mouth ulcers, sore throats and vaginal thrush. Take 15 drops, 3 times daily, in a little water about half an hour before meals. People suffering from HIV or Leukaemia should consult a Healthcare Professional before using this product.

KAVA-KAVA

This fresh herbal tincture is made from the root of the Kava-Kava, which belongs to the Pepper family and is found in nearly all the Pacific Islands. It is non-addictive but its excellent sedative and 'calming' qualities have proved beneficial in cases of headache, mouth ulcers, and stress. Take 20 drops in a little water twice daily. Long term use of this product is not recommended and after 4 weeks use you should have at least one weeks break. If you are taking prescribed tranquillisers or medication for epilepsy you should seek medical advice before using this product. Do not take Kava-Kava at the same time as alcohol. It could increase the effects of barbiturates, anti-depressants and sedatives. You may feel a slight numbing sensation in the mouth when you use this tincture but this can be minimised by diluting the tincture well in water and drinking quickly. Not suitable for children.

ELEUTHEROCOCCUS

This fresh herbal tincture of Eleutherococcus senticosus or Siberian Ginseng has been used for thousands of years to help the body adapt to mental and physical stress. Various studies have shown that this herb can help the body deal with fatigue and mental tiredness and so 'keep going'. Take 20 drops twice daily in a little water to help allergies, concentration and stress. If you are taking prescribed medication for nervous or heart disorders, diabetes, oral contraceptives or HRT, or if you suffer from high blood pressure or schizophrenia, you should consult a practitioner before using this herb.

If you choose to, you could also take the following in supplementation:

BETA-CAROTENE – 2,500 IU daily should help reduce catarrh, frequent colds/flu, cystitis, eczema, headaches, mouth ulcers and sore throats.

VITAMIN B2 – 100mg daily has proved beneficial in treating eczema and mouth ulcers.

VITAMIN B6 – 100mg twice daily is very useful if you are suffering from headaches.

VITAMIN B12 – 50 micrograms daily can bring relief to mouth ulcers.

BIOFLAVONOIDS – 100mg twice daily taken with Vitamin C, will increase your resistance to colds and flu.

VITAMIN C – 500mg twice daily. Everybody's essential vitamin which is especially helpful for catarrh, frequent colds/flu, cystitis, eczema, mouth ulcers, sore throats and vaginal thrush.

EVENING PRIMROSE OIL – 500mg daily to be taken with care if you have ever had epilepsy. It can help reduce catarrh and eczema.

FOLIC ACID – 100-200 micrograms daily should help fatigue/ mouth ulcers.

GARLIC – 300mg daily taken as a supplement and used in cooking to reduce catarrh, frequent colds/flu and fatigue.

IRON – 15mg daily. The small amount included in a multi-vitamin should be enough to help mouth ulcers.

MAGNESIUM – 100-300mg daily can often reduce headaches.

POTASSIUM – 100mg daily, taken in a multi-vitamin, will often alleviate a headache.

SELENIUM – When used in a shampoo, it relieves eczema of the scalp.

ZINC – 10-15mg twice daily. One of the most important minerals. It can help frequent colds/flu, eczema headaches, mouth ulcers and sore throats.

WHAT TO TAKE AND WHY
GROUP C

If your highest score has occurred in Group C, you should find relief by taking the following three items:

GINKGO BILOBA

Ginkgo biloba has been used for years in China for improving the memory, where it is known as the 'memory tree'. It has been shown to improve the cerebral circulation and is useful for the prevention of strokes and transient ischaemic attacks. For patients in Group C it can also be used for concentration, depression, headaches, memory loss, varicose veins. Take 15 drops in half a glass of water, three times daily before meals.

MOLKOSAN

Molkosan is produced from fresh Alpine Whey by a natural fermentation process which conserves all the goodness and nourishment of the contents of the whey. Patients in this group should find it helpful for nail problems, oral thrush and sore throats. For internal use take 1 teaspoonful to a glass of mineral water three times daily before or with meals.

KAVA-KAVA

This fresh herbal tincture is made from the root of the Kava-Kava, which belongs to the Pepper family and is found in nearly all the Pacific Islands. It is non-addictive but for patients in this group its excellent sedative and 'calming' qualities should prove beneficial in cases of headache, memory loss and mouth ulcers. Take 20 drops in a little water twice daily. Long term use of this product is not recommended and after 4 weeks use you should have at least one weeks break. If you are taking prescribed tranquillisers or medication for epilepsy you should seek medical advice before using this product. Do not take Kava-Kava at the same time as alcohol. It could increase the effects of barbiturates, anti-depressants and sedatives. You may feel a slight numbing sensation in the mouth when you use this tincture but this can be minimised by diluting the tincture well in water and drinking quickly. Not suitable for children.

If you choose to, you could also take the following in supplementation:

BETA-CAROTENE – 2,500 IU daily, should help poor hair, headaches and eye problems.

VITAMIN B1 – 100mg daily, taken with other B vitamins, can ease depression.

VITAMIN B6 – 100mg twice daily is very useful if you are suffering from depression and headaches.

VITAMIN C – 500mg twice daily Everybody's essential vitamin, especially helpful for depression, eye problems and oral thrush.

CALCIUM – 1,000 mg daily will often reduce the frequency of dandruff.

EVENING PRIMROSE OIL – 500mg daily (to be taken with care if you have ever had epilepsy) can help improve circulation and reduce dandruff.

GARLIC – 300mg daily taken as a supplement and used in cooking to improve memory and reduce wind.

MAGNESIUM – 100-300mg daily can often reduce headaches.

POTASSIUM – 100mg daily, taken in a multi-vitamin, will often alleviate a headache and improve memory loss.

SELENIUM – when used in a shampoo is great to relieve dandruff.

ZINC – 10-15mg twice daily – One of the most important minerals, it can help reduce dandruff and depression, improve circulation and memory.

WHAT TO TAKE AND WHY
GROUP D

If your highest score has occurred in Group D, you should find relief by taking the following three items:

MOLKOSAN

Molkosan is produced from fresh Alpine Whey by a natural fermentation process which conserves all the goodness and nourishment of the contents of the whey. Patients in this group should find it helpful for eczema, oral thrush, skin problems, and vaginal thrush

For internal use take 1 teaspoonful to a glass of mineral water three times daily before or with meals. For external use apply to small wounds, abrasions and skin rashes either neat or, if this produces a stinging sensation, diluted in a ratio of 1:4 with water. For insect bites, apply undiluted. As a gargle mix one tablespoon Molkosan to four tablespoons water and gargle three times daily. As a vaginal douche mix 2 teaspoonfuls in half a teacup water. You should be able to obtain a douche kit from any good chemist. For a hair and body rinse dilute Molkosan 1:10 with water and rinse hair and skin after showers, then towel dry. Do not rinse again.

GINKGO BILOBA

Ginkgo biloba has been used for years in China for improving the memory, where it is known as the 'memory tree'. It has been shown to improve the cerebral circulation and is useful for the prevention of strokes and transient ischaemic attacks. For patients in Group D it can also be used for circulation problems, eye problems and headaches. Take 15 drops in half a glass of water, three times daily before meals.

BLACK COHOSH

This fresh herbal extract comes from the root of a member of the Buttercup family originally called Squaw Root by North American Indians because of its 'normalising' and relaxing effects on the female reproductive system. It has a natural source of salicylic acid that helps reduce inflammation and pain. It should prove beneficial for patients in this group suffering from menopausal problems, period pains, and PMT.

Take 20 drops in a little water twice daily, about half an hour before meals. Patients who are allergic to aspirin should not use this product.

If you choose to, you could also take the following in capsule or tablet form.

BETA-CAROTENE – 2,500 IU daily should help reduce allergies, eczema, eye problems and headaches.

VITAMIN B2 – 100mg daily has proved beneficial in treating eczema.

VITAMIN B6 – 100mg twice daily is very useful if you are suffering from headaches.

BIOFLAVONOIDS – 100mg twice daily taken with Vitamin C, will help to increase your resistance to allergies.

VITAMIN C – 500mg twice daily. Everybody's essential vitamin, especially helpful for aches and pains, allergies, eczema, eye problems, oral thrush and vaginal thrush.

CALCIUM – 1,000 mg daily should ease aches, pains and allergies.

VITAMIN E – 400 IU daily. Often called 'the circulation vitamin' it should also help reduce diarrhoea and eczema.

EVENING PRIMROSE OIL – 500mg daily, (to be taken with care if you have ever had epilepsy,) can help reduce allergies, circulation, diarrhoea and eczema.

GARLIC – 300mg daily taken as a supplement and used in cooking to reduce wind.

MAGNESIUM – 100-300mg daily can often reduce muscular aches and pains, and headaches.

POTASSIUM – at least 100mg daily, taken in a multivitamin, will often alleviate a headache.

SELENIUM – when used in a shampoo is great to relieve eczema of the scalp.

ZINC – 10-15mg twice daily. One of the most important minerals, it can help eczema, headaches and oral thrush.

WHAT TO TAKE AND WHY
GROUP E

If your highest score has occurred in Group E, you should find relief by taking the following three items:

URTICALCIN

This is a combination of Homoeopathic preparations. It is used where a lack of calcium is indicated such as catarrh, coeliac disease, colds, eczema, fatigue, insomnia and psoriasis. Take three tablets, twice daily, allowing them to dissolve slowly under the tongue. For maximum benefit this product should be taken for at least two months.

KAVA–KAVA

This fresh herbal tincture is made from the root of the Kava–Kava, which belongs to the Pepper family and is found in nearly all the Pacific Islands. It is non-addictive but for patients in this group its excellent sedative and 'calming' qualities should prove beneficial in cases of headache, insomnia, memory loss, muscle pain and stress. Take 20 drops in a little water twice daily. For insomnia, take 30 drops in water, about an hour before bedtime. Long term use of this product is not recommended and after 4 weeks use you should have at least one weeks break. If you are taking prescribed tranquillisers or medication for epilepsy you should seek medical advice before using this product. Do not take Kava–Kava at the same time as alcohol. It could increase the effects of barbiturates, anti-depressants and sedatives. You may feel a slight numbing sensation in the mouth when you use this tincture but this can be minimised by diluting the tincture well in water and drinking quickly. Not suitable for children.

MOLKOSAN

Molkosan is produced from fresh Alpine Whey by a natural fermentation process which conserves all the goodness and nourishment of the contents of the whey. Patients in this group should find it helpful for catarrh, eczema, frequent colds/flu, psoriasis, sore throats and skin problems, For internal use take 1 teaspoonful to a glass of mineral water three times daily before or with meals. For external use apply to small wounds, abrasions and skin rashes either neat or, if this produces a stinging sensation, diluted in a ratio of 1:4 with water. For insect bites, apply undiluted. As a gargle mix one tablespoon Molkosan to four tablespoons water and gargle three times daily.

If you choose to, you could also take the following in capsule or tablet form.

BETA-CAROTENE – 2,500 IU daily should help reduce catarrh, frequent colds/flu, eczema, headaches and psoriasis.

VITAMIN B2 – 100mg daily has proved beneficial in treating eczema.

VITAMIN B3 – 100mg daily taken with other B vitamins can help improve sleeping problems

VITAMIN B6 – 100mg twice daily is very useful if you are suffering from headaches or sleeping problems.

BIOFLAVONOIDS – 100mg twice daily taken with Vitamin C, will increase your resistance to colds and flu.

VITAMIN C – 500mg twice daily. Everybody's essential vitamin, especially helpful for aches and pains, catarrh, frequent colds/flu, eczema and psoriasis.

CALCIUM – 1,000 mg daily should help to ease aches and pains, and sleeping problems.

VITAMIN E – 400 IU – Often called 'the circulation vitamin' it should also help reduce the frequency of colds/flu, diarrhoea and eczema.

EVENING PRIMROSE OIL – 500mg daily, (to be taken with care if you have ever had epilepsy,) can help reduce catarrh, diarrhoea, eczema and psoriasis.

FOLIC ACID – 100-200 micrograms daily should help fatigue and sleeping problems.

GARLIC – 300mg daily taken as a supplement and used in cooking to reduce catarrh, frequent colds/flu and fatigue.

MAGNESIUM – 100-300mg daily can reduce general aches and pains, headaches and sleeping problems.

POTASSIUM – 100mg daily, taken in a multivitamin, will often alleviate a headache.

SELENIUM – when used in a shampoo is great to relieve eczema of the scalp.

ZINC – 10-15mg daily. One of the most important minerals, it can help breast tenderness, frequent colds/flu, eczema, headaches and psoriasis.

WHAT TO TAKE AND WHY GROUP F

If your highest score has occurred in Group F, you should find relief by taking the following three items:

MOLKOSAN

Molkosan is produced from fresh Alpine Whey by a natural fermentation process which conserves all the goodness and nourishment of the contents of the whey. Patients in this group should find it helpful for anal irritation, athletes foot, catarrh, eczema, nail problems, psoriasis, sore throats, For internal use take 1 teaspoonful to a glass of mineral water three times daily before or with meals. For external use apply to small wounds, abrasions and skin rashes either neat or, if this produces a stinging sensation, diluted in a ratio of 1:4 with water. For insect bites, apply undiluted. For a hair and body rinse dilute Molkosan 1:10 with water and rinse hair and skin after showers, then towel dry. Do not rinse again.

UVA-URSI COMPLEX

This combination of herbs has been formulated to relieve the symptoms associated with urinary tract infections. It should prove beneficial to patients suffering from bedwetting, cystitis or incontinence. Take 15 drops twice daily in a little water about half an hour before meals. If symptoms persist for more than one week, if you have a fever or there is blood in the urine you should consult a practitioner. You should not take Uva-ursi Complex if you are pregnant or breastfeeding. Solidago Complex should be taken instead if you suffer from cystitis during pregnancy.

KELP TABLETS

This is a natural, pure Pacific ocean algae (kelp) derivative in tablet form as a natural supplement to help your thyroid. It should also help patients in Group F suffering from breast tenderness, constipation, fatigue, and muscle pain. Take one tablet morning and noon before meals. *DO NOT TAKE AFTER TEATIME*. This product should not be taken by anyone with high blood pressure, kidney disorders or thyroid conditions, unless under medical supervision. You should not take Kelp tablets if you are taking Thyroxine or if you are allergic to iodine.

If you choose to, you could also take the following in supplementation:

BETA-CAROTENE – 2,500 IU daily should help reduce catarrh, cystitis, eczema, psoriasis and sore throats and improve poor hair.

VITAMIN B2 – 100mg daily has proved beneficial in treating eczema.

VITAMIN B6 – 100mg twice daily is very useful if you are suffering from breast tenderness.

VITAMIN C – 500mg twice daily. Everybody's essential vitamin, especially helpful for aches and pains, breast tenderness, catarrh, constipation, cystitis, eczema, psoriasis and sore throats.

CALCIUM – 1,000 mg daily can help to relieve aches, pains and dandruff.

VITAMIN E – 400 IU daily Often called 'the circulation vitamin' it should also help reduce cystitis and eczema.

EVENING PRIMROSE OIL – 500mg daily to be taken with care if you have ever had epilepsy. It can help reduce breast tenderness, catarrh and dandruff.

GARLIC – 300mg daily taken as a supplement and used in cooking to reduce catarrh.

MAGNESIUM – 100-300mg daily can reduce aches, pains and constipation.

SELENIUM – when used in a shampoo is great to relieve dandruff and eczema of the scalp.

ZINC – 10-15mg twice daily. One of the most important minerals, it can help breast tenderness, eczema, nail problems, psoriasis and sore throats.

WHAT TO TAKE AND WHY
GROUP G

If your highest score has occurred in Group G, you should find relief by taking the following three items:

WHEAT GERM OIL CAPSULES
Vitamin E found in the wheat germ oil influences the function of the muscles and gonadal system. It may be necessary to take this for a few months before any benefit is noticed, but patients in Group G should find it helps breast tenderness, dandruff, depression, digestion, irritability, light, irregular or painful periods and memory loss. Take 1 capsule, 3 times daily. Gluten is a protein, but wheat germ oil is a fatty acid so even those with a gluten allergy generally tolerate this product very well.

VALERIANA OFFICINALIS
This fresh herbal preparation is used as a natural calmative and patients in this group should find it helps with problems pertaining to sleep disturbances and the nervous system also headaches, insomnia, muscle pain, period pain, stomach cramps, stress, tension and wind. Take 10 drops in a little water, three times daily. For cases of insomnia take 30 drops in a little water about half an hour before going to bed at night. Not recommended for pregnancy or nursing mothers without medical supervision.

BLACK COHOSH
This fresh herbal extract comes from the root of a member of the Buttercup family originally called Squaw Root by North American Indians because of its 'normalising' and relaxing effects on the female reproductive system. It has a natural source of salicylic acid that helps reduce inflammation and pain. It should prove beneficial for patients in this group suffering from arthritis, hot flushes, and menopausal problems, period pains, and pmt

Take 20 drops in a little water twice daily, about half an hour before meals. Patients who are allergic to aspirin should not use this product.

If you choose to, you could also take the following in supplementation

BETA-CAROTENE – 2,500 IU daily should help reduce allergies and headaches, and improve poor hair.

VITAMIN B1 – 100mg daily taken with other B vitamins, can ease depression.

VITAMIN B3 – 100mg daily taken with other B vitamins, can help sleeping problems.

VITAMIN B6 – 100mg twice daily is very useful if you are suffering from breast tenderness, depression, and headaches or sleeping problems.

BIOFLAVONOIDS – 100mg twice daily taken with Vitamin C, will often reduce allergies.

VITAMIN C – 500mg twice daily. Everybody's essential vitamin, especially helpful for allergies, breast tenderness, constipation and depression.

CALCIUM – 1,000 mg daily can help to reduce allergies, dandruff and sleeping problems.

EVENING PRIMROSE OIL – 500mg daily (to be taken with care if you have ever had epilepsy) can help reduce allergies, breast tenderness and dandruff.

FOLIC ACID – 100-200 micrograms daily should help you to sleep.

GARLIC – 300mg daily taken as a supplement and used in cooking to improve memory and reduce wind.

MAGNESIUM – 100-300mg daily can reduce breast tenderness, constipation, headaches and sleeping problems.

POTASSIUM – at least 100mg daily, taken in a multivitamin, will often alleviate a headache and improve memory loss.

SELENIUM – when used in a shampoo is great to relieve dandruff.

ZINC – 10-15mg taken twice daily. One of the most important minerals, it can help breast tenderness, depression and headaches.

WHAT TO TAKE AND WHY
GROUP H

If your highest score has occurred in Group H, you should find relief by taking the following three items:

ECHINACEA TINCTURE

This is a 'natural antibiotic' which is considered to be the prime herbal remedy for the immune system. In Group H patients it has proved extremely beneficial, in cases of allergies, anal irritation, eye problems, fatigue, frequent colds/flu, oral thrush, skin disorders, sore throats, and vaginal thrush. Take 15 drops, 3 times daily, in a little water about half an hour before meals. People suffering from HIV or Leukaemia should consult a Healthcare Professional before using this product.

KELP TABLETS

This is a natural, pure Pacific ocean algae (kelp) derivative in tablet form as a natural supplement to help your thyroid. It should also help patients in Group H suffering from allergies, breast tenderness, constipation, fatigue, and muscle pain. Take one tablet morning and noon before meals. *DO NOT TAKE AFTER TEATIME.* This product should not be taken by anyone with high blood pressure, kidney disorders or thyroid conditions, unless under medical supervision. You should not take Kelp tablets if you are taking Thyroxine or if you are allergic to iodine.

BLACK COHOSH

This fresh herbal extract comes from the root of a member of the Buttercup family originally called Squaw Root by North American Indians because of its 'normalising' and relaxing effects on the female reproductive system. It has a natural source of salicylic acid that helps reduce inflammation and pain. It should prove beneficial for patients in this group suffering from arthritis, hot flushes, and menopausal problems, period pains, and PMT. Take 20 drops in a little water twice daily, about half an hour before meals. Patients who are allergic to aspirin should not use this product.

If you choose to, you could also take the following in supplementation:

BETA-CAROTENE – 2,500 IU daily should help reduce allergies, frequent colds/flu, eye problems and sore throats.

VITAMIN B1 – 100mg daily taken with other B vitamins, can ease depression.

VITAMIN B6 – 100mg twice daily is very useful if you are suffering from depression.

BIOFLAVONOIDS – 100mg three times daily taken with Vitamin C, will often reduce allergies and increase your resistance to colds and flu.

VITAMIN C – 500mg twice daily. Everybody's essential vitamin, especially helpful for aches and pains, allergies, frequent colds/flu, constipation, depression, eye problems, oral thrush, sore throats and vaginal thrush.

CALCIUM – 1,000 mg daily can help to reduce general aches and pains.

VITAMIN E – 400 IU daily Often called 'the circulation vitamin' it should also help reduce the frequency of colds/flu.

EVENING PRIMROSE OIL – 500mg daily (to be taken with care if you have ever had epilepsy) can help reduce allergies.

FOLIC ACID – 100-200 micrograms daily should ease fatigue.

GARLIC – 300mg daily taken as a supplement and used in cooking to reduce frequent colds/flu and fatigue.

MAGNESIUM – 100-300mg daily can reduce aches, pains and constipation.

ZINC – 10-15mg taken twice daily. One of the most important minerals, it can help frequent colds/flu, depression, oral thrush and sore throats.

WHAT TO TAKE AND WHY
GROUP J

If your highest score has occurred in Group J, you should find relief by taking the following three items:

ECHINACEA TINCTURE

This is a 'natural antibiotic' which is considered to be the prime herbal remedy for the immune system. In Group J patients it has proved extremely beneficial, in more stubborn cases of cystitis, diarrhoea, fatigue, frequent colds/flu, nail problems, oral thrush and sore throats. Take 15 drops, 3 times daily, in a little water about half an hour before meals. People suffering from HIV or Leukaemia should consult a Healthcare Professional before using this product.

ELEUTHEROCOCCUS

This fresh herbal tincture of Eleutherococcus senticosus or Siberian Ginseng has been used for thousands of years to help the body adapt to mental and physical stress. Various studies have shown that this herb can help the body deal with fatigue and mental tiredness and so 'keep going'. Take 20 drops twice daily in a little water to help allergies, concentration and stress. If you are taking prescribed medication for nervous or heart disorders, diabetes, oral contraceptives or HRT, or if you suffer from high blood pressure or schizophrenia, you should consult a practitioner before using this herb.

VALERIANA OFFICINALIS

This fresh herbal preparation is used as a natural calmative and patients in this group should find it helps with problems pertaining to stress, sleep disturbances and the nervous system also insomnia. Take 10 drops in a little water, three times daily. For cases of insomnia take 30 drops in a little water about half an hour before going to bed at night. Not recommended for pregnancy or nursing mothers without medical supervision.

If you choose to, you could also take the following in supplementation:

BETA-CAROTENE – 2,500 IU daily should help reduce frequent colds/flu, cystitis, mouth ulcers and sore throats.

VITAMIN B2 – 100mg daily has proved beneficial in treating mouth ulcers.

VITAMIN B3 – 100mg daily when taken with other 'B' vitamins, can help improve sleeping problems

VITAMIN B6 – 100mg twice daily is very useful if you are suffering from sleeping problems.

VITAMIN B12 – 50 micrograms daily can bring relief to mouth ulcers

BIOFLAVONOIDS – 100mg twice daily taken with Vitamin C, will often increase your resistance to colds and flu.

VITAMIN C – 500mg twice daily. Everybody's essential vitamin which is especially helpful for frequent colds/flu, cystitis, mouth ulcers, oral thrush and sore throats.

CALCIUM – 1,000 mg daily can help to improve sleeping.

VITAMIN E – 400 IU daily. Often called 'the circulation vitamin' it should also help reduce the frequency of colds/flu, cystitis and diarrhoea.

EVENING PRIMROSE OIL – 500mg daily (to be taken with care if you have ever had epilepsy) can help improve diarrhoea.

FOLIC ACID – 100-200 micrograms daily should help fatigue, mouth ulcers and sleeping problems.

GARLIC – 300mg daily taken as a supplement and used in cooking to reduce frequent colds/flu and fatigue.

IRON – 15mg daily the small amount contained in a multivitamin should be enough to help mouth ulcers.

MAGNESIUM – 100-300mg daily can reduce sleeping problems.

ZINC – 10-15mg taken twice daily. One of the most important minerals, it can help frequent colds/flu, mouth ulcers, nail problems, oral thrush and sore throats.

WHAT TO TAKE AND WHY
GROUP K

If your highest score has occurred in Group K, you should find relief by taking the following three items:

GINKGO BILOBA
Ginkgo biloba has been used for years in China for improving the memory, where it is known as the 'memory tree'. It has been shown to improve the cerebral circulation and is useful for the prevention of strokes and transient ischaemic attacks. For patients in Group K it can also help circulation problems, concentration, depression, eye problems, headaches and memory loss. Take 15 drops in half a glass of water, three times daily before meals.

VIOLA TRICOLOR
This fresh extract of Viola tricolor, commonly found in Europe, is famous for its cleansing action, which can be beneficial to many skin conditions. It helps to eliminate toxins by increasing the blood flow to the kidneys and its gentle action makes it suitable for adults and children. Adults should take 15 drops in a little water, twice daily. Children 7-10 drops in a little water twice daily, and infants up to 3-5 drops in a little water, twice daily. You should not take this product during pregnancy without medical supervision.

PEPPERMINT COMPLEX
This fresh herb tincture is a mixture of peppermint, fennel, centaury, tormentil and liquorice that combine to help digestive function and improve the symptoms of Irritable Bowel Syndrome. Patients in this group should find it helps depression, indigestion, nausea, stress and wind. Take 15 drops in a little water, twice daily, about half an hour before meals.

Not to be given to children unless under medical supervision.

As this product contains a very small amount of liquorice, (5%) it is advisable to seek medical advice if you are also taking medication for hypertension or diabetes. Peppermint Complex should not be taken during pregnancy.

If you choose to, you could also take the following in supplementation

BETA-CAROTENE – 2,500 IU daily should help reduce eczema, eye problems, headaches and psoriasis.

VITAMIN B1 – 100mg daily, taken with other B vitamins, can ease depression.

VITAMIN B2 – 100mg daily has proved beneficial in treating eczema.

VITAMIN B6 – 100mg twice daily is very useful if you are suffering from depression or headaches.

VITAMIN C – 500mg twice daily Everybody's essential vitamin, especially helpful for depression, eczema, eye problems and psoriasis.

VITAMIN E – 400 IU daily often called 'the circulation vitamin' it should also help eczema.

EVENING PRIMROSE OIL – 500mg daily (to be taken with care if you have ever had epilepsy). It can help improve circulation and reduce eczema and psoriasis.

FOLIC ACID – 100-200 micrograms daily should help fatigue.

GARLIC – 300mg daily taken as a supplement and used in cooking to improve memory and reduce fatigue and wind.

MAGNESIUM – 100-300mg daily can often reduce headaches.

POTASSIUM – at least 100mg daily, taken in a multivitamin, will often alleviate a headache and improve memory loss.

SELENIUM – when used in a shampoo is great to relieve eczema of the scalp.

ZINC – 10-15mg taken twice daily. One of the most important minerals, it can help depression, eczema, headaches and psoriasis

DIETARY GUIDELINES

The most important thing in treating Candida is to stick to the diet. If you do not follow the strict yeast and sugar free diet while you are undergoing treatment you will never win the battle against this condition.

Don't have any fruit in the early stages of treatment because all fruit, (including tomatoes) contains natural sugar; also avoid honey and sugar substitutes such as lactose, maltose, mannitol, natural sweetener, raw sugar, saccharine, sorbitol, sucrose, syrup, turbinado, E420, E421.

When leaving out forbidden foods, some people may feel worse for a few days. This is known as a *yeast die-off* and is a good sign; you can almost regard it as a withdrawal symptom. It requires total commitment and discipline by the patient to achieve the best and longest lasting results.

If you are a vegetarian, or even if you are not, I suggest you substitute the meat content of the recipes with one of the many brands of protein substitute available. Never be afraid to experiment with something new – provided it is on your diet sheet. If you are a dedicated carnivore then I suggest you do as I did which is to think when you are eating – are you actually enjoying the taste of the meat, or are you enjoying the sauce or the way in which it was cooked? If it's the former, then you are probably beyond all help! If, like me, you find you are really enjoying the sauce, then LEAVE MEAT ALONE and stack up on those veggies! There are lots of other ways to get your protein.

A big concern to us all is Genetically Modified Food. This really is a political 'hot potato' but until a government or the World Health Organisation can guarantee 100% that it has no long term side effects I suggest you avoid it like the plague. Make sure you read the labels on everything you buy. Wherever possible ensure the things you eat are organically grown, better still find a space in the garden to grow things yourself then they will go straight from the ground into your cooking pot with no delay. Delicious.

In the early stages some people say, "The diet is hard", but the diet is no worse than you let it be. View it as a challenge and tackle it with enthusiasm knowing it will help to make you well again. You will be amazed how many of your usual recipes you can adapt, in fact many people feel so well on the first stage that they stay on it permanently.

Remember that herbs and spices, in moderation, are your best friends. Sadly too many people, when they see the word 'diet', think *'lettuce leaf'* but this is **not** a slimming diet, it is a diet for people with a specific health problem.

It is possible you will loose weight because many people with a Candida overgrowth have a weight problem. The strange thing is, if you are underweight, you will probably put weight on when following this regime. The body is a wonderful machine and, when given the correct nutrients and allowed to function properly, will usually balance itself out.

EVERYONE IS DIFFERENT. Some people need to be on the first stage of the diet for a month, some are on it for six months or a year. I would suggest a month as the minimum amount of time to follow each stage of treatment.

The first stage of the diet is the hardest as it is virtually detoxification. At the end of your first month, don't be tempted to go wading on in to Stage 2, throwing caution to the wind and hang the consequences.

Look back over the questionnaires and see if your original problems have gone, or almost gone. If more than two problems remain, even if only slightly, you should stay on Stage 1 for another month at least.

When you feel you have improved sufficiently to progress to Stage Two – BE CAREFUL. Never re-introduce more than one 'new' food a day. If any of your old symptoms return, stop and think, "What have I eaten in the last twenty-four hours that I have not eaten for a month or so?"

Wait for four days, and then try the doubtful food again. If your symptoms return you will know you are allergic to that specific food and should avoid it.

After at least a month on Stage 2, wait until there are no symptoms as you did before, then reintroduce the foods given for Stage 3, and so on.

Off you go – good luck!

STAGE 1 DIET & RECIPES

CHOOSE AS MUCH AS YOU WANT FROM ANY OF THE FOLLOWING ITEMS, BUT STICK TO THESE ITEMS ONLY. REMEMBER – IF IT IS NOT ON THE LIST, YOU CAN'T HAVE IT!

VEGETABLES – Alfalfa sprouts, Artichoke (Chinese), Asparagus, Aubergine, Bamboo Shoots, Bean Sprouts, Broccoli, Cabbages, Cauliflower, Carrots, Celery, Celeriac, Chicory, Chinese Cabbage, Courgettes, Cucumber, Curly Cress, Endive, Fennel, Garlic, Gherkin, Green Pepper, Haricot Beans, Kale, Kelp, Kohlrabi, Leek, Lettuce, Onion, Okra, Parsnip, Potato, Pumpkin, Rape, Radish, Red Pepper, Sea Kale, Shallot, String Bean, Turnip tops, Watercress

HERBS & SPICES – Allspice, Anise, Apple Mint, Basil, Black Pepper, Borage, Caraway, Cardamom, Chervil, Chive, Clove, Coriander, Cumin, Curry Powder, Dill, Fenugreek, Ginger, Horseradish, Lovage. Mace, Marjoram, Mint, Nutmeg, Oregano, Paprika, Parsley, Peppercorns, Peppermint, Pimento, Rosemary, Saffron, Sage, Salt, Savory, Sorrel, Spearmint, Tarragon, Thyme, Turmeric

FOWL – *NOT BREADED, BATTERED OR SERVED IN READY MADE SAUCE* – Chicken and Chicken eggs, Duck and Duck eggs, Goose and Goose eggs, Pheasant, Pigeon, Partridge, Quail, Turkey and Turkey eggs

SEAFOOD – *NOT BREADED, BATTERED OR SERVED IN READY MADE SAUCE* –
Abalone, Clam, Cockle, Crab, Lobster, Mussel, Oyster, Prawn, Scallop, Shrimp, Squid

MEAT – Lamb, Rabbit – or substitute with a myco-protein

FISH – *NOT BREADED, BATTERED OR SERVED IN READY-MADE SAUCE. TINNED FISH MUST BE IN OIL OR BRINE* –
 Anchovy, Carp, Caviar (roe), Chub, Eel, Flounder, Herring, Mackerel, Salmon, Sole, Sprats, Plaice, Pike, Pollock, Tuna, Trout, Whitebait

GRAINS – Barley, Brown rice, Oats, Rye, Wild rice *NOTE*: Barley and Oats are usually safe unless you have a gluten allergy. If this is the case avoid these until Stage 4

MISCELLANEOUS – Butter (in small quantities), Cottage cheese, Herbal teas, Oat flakes, Olive oil, Pumpkin seeds, Safflower oil, Sea salt, Sunflower seed and oil, Soda bread, Spring water, Wholemeal pasta, Wholemeal flour, Yeast free crispbread (read the labels carefully) Natural live yoghurt. *NOTE*: Oat flakes, Wholemeal pasta and Wholemeal flour are usually safe unless you have a gluten allergy. If this is so you should avoid these until Stage 4

You must NOT have – Anything that is not on this list, which includes sugar in all its forms, (including sweeteners). Sweeteners are often 'disguised' under the following names, or 'E' numbers: Acesulfame Potassium, Aspartame, Dextrose, Fructose, Galactose, Glucose syrup, Isomalt, Lactose, Maltose, Mannitol, Sorbitol, Sucrose, E420, E421.

Avoid anything containing yeast, or yeast extracts such as Marmite, Bovril etc., or mushrooms, (read all labels very carefully). Anything containing processed fat, food colouring or additives, 'junk' foods, milk and milk products, except natural yoghurt.

Avoid fruit of any kind, including tomatoes and ANYTHING that has been genetically modified.

Instead of ordinary tea, drink herb tea and instead of coffee drink a coffee substitute such as Bambu.

POTAGE PARMENTIER   Serves 4

Ingredients:
>2-3 leeks
>1lb/450g potatoes
>2oz/50g butter
>20fl.oz/550ml water
>1 egg yolk

Prepare and cut the leeks and potatoes and fry lightly in the butter for 5 minutes.
Cover with water and simmer until vegetables are tender.
Sieve the soup, add more water depending on the consistency required, and bring to the boil.
Skim the soup and beat in the egg yolk. Serve at once.

WATERCRESS SOUP   Serves 1

Ingredients:
>1 medium potato, diced
>1 onion, diced
>1 leek, diced
>Black pepper
>Sea salt
>15fl.oz/425ml vegetable stock
>1 bunch watercress, washed and trimmed

Place potato, onion, leek, salt and pepper and 5 fl.oz/150ml of stock into a saucepan with lid. Cook on top of the stove for 10 minutes on moderate heat, stirring occasionally.
Add watercress and the rest of the stock, cover and simmer for a further 10-15 minutes, until vegetables are soft.
Remove from heat and liquidise.
Return to pan and reheat prior to serving.

WARMING WINTER SOUP   Serves 4

Ingredients:

     1oz/30g long grain brown rice
     40fl.oz/1litre chicken stock
     4 carrots, scraped and thickly sliced
     2 large onions, peeled and sliced
     1 clove garlic, crushed
     1 red pepper, diced and de-seeded
     2 tblsp chopped parsley
     Seasoning

Put rice in a pan with chicken stock, carrots, onions, garlic and seasoning and simmer for 20 minutes.
Add red pepper and parsley.
Simmer for a further 10 minutes. Serve.

POTATO SOUP WITH OATMEAL   Serves 4

Ingredients:

     1 teacup oatmeal
     7 teacups cold water
     1 onion, chopped
     1 tsp mixed herbs
     Salt and pepper to taste
     5 or 6 medium potatoes, peeled and diced

Cook oatmeal in water until fairly soft.
Add diced potato, seasoning, mixed herbs and onion. Boil until thick and creamy.
Simmer for 2 hours.

BARLEY CHICKEN SOUP   Serves 4

Ingredients:

      3lbs/1.5kg jointed chicken
      70fl.oz/2litres water
      4oz/100g chopped onion
      1 tblsp sea salt
      4oz/100g barley
      8oz/225g chopped celery

Place all ingredients in a large pan and cook over a medium heat until everything is tender.
Remove all chicken bones. Liquidise, reheat and serve.
NOTE: May be cooked all day in a slow cooker.

SEAFOOD SPAGHETTI   Serves 4

Ingredients:

      6oz/175g wholemeal spaghetti
      1 tblsp olive oil
      1oz/30g butter
      4oz/100g courgettes
      2 egg yolks
      4oz/100g prawns
      1 small carton yoghurt
      Parsley for garnish

Cook spaghetti in boiling water for 10-12 minutes.
Heat oil and butter in frying pan, add sliced courgettes and cook over moderate heat for 5-10 minutes.
Half way through cooking time, place prawns in a small pan and mix with egg yolks and add yoghurt. Warm gently.
Drain spaghetti and combine with courgettes and prawn mix.
Garnish with parsley if desired.

PLAICE AND PRAWN PARCELS   Serves 4

Ingredients:

    4 plaice fillets, each about 5oz/150g
    8oz/225g peeled prawns
    1 lemon

Put each plaice fillet on a long sheet of foil.
Cover each fillet with 2oz/50g prawns and a squeeze of lemon.
Fold up foil to make a parcel.
Put all 4 parcels in a baking tray and bake at 350F, 180C, Gas Mark 4 for 20–30 minutes
Serve with a lettuce and watercress salad.

GRILLED PLAICE SURPRISE   Serves 4

Ingredients:

    1 tsp dried basil
    Grated rind and juice of 1 lemon
    ¼tsp garlic granules
    4 plaice fillets
    Watercress to garnish

Mix together dried basil, grated rind and juice of 1 lemon, and garlic granules.
Arrange plaice fillets on a grill pan and brush with lemon mixture.
Grill until tender, brushing with any remaining lemon mixture during cooking.
Garnish with lemon twists and watercress before serving.

FISH CAKES   Serves 4

Ingredients:

> 1lb/450g cooked white fish
> 8oz/225g cooked brown rice
> 1 egg
> 1 small onion, finely chopped
> 1 tblsp lemon juice
> 8oz/225g soda bread crumbs.
> 3 tblsp melted butter

Beat Egg. Add fish, rice, onion, lemon juice and oil.
Blend well and form into 8 patties.
Roll in soda bread crumbs and place on a lightly oiled baking sheet.
Bake in oven at 350F, 180C, Gas Mark 4 for about 15 minutes until brown and
bubbly.

FISH BROCHETTES   Serves 4

Ingredients:

> 8oz/225g boned white fish in large chunks
> 12 large prawns
> 2 courgettes
> 4 slices lemon
> 2 tblsp lemon juice
> Salt and pepper to taste
> 2 tblsp olive oil

Cut fish into large chunks. Place in shallow dish and sprinkle with lemon juice
and oil. Chill for 1 hour.
Trim and slice 2 courgettes.
Cut lemon slices in half to make 8 half slices.
Remove head, tail and shells from prawns.
Thread fish, lemon, courgettes and prawns onto four skewers and brush with
any remaining lemon juice and oil.
Cook under a preheated grill for 10 minutes until fish is just cooked. Season
well before serving.

DILL FISH FILLETS   Serves 4

Ingredients:

  4 x 6oz/175g skinned white fish fillets
  4 tsp dried or 2 tblsp fresh chopped dill
  1oz/30g butter
  Salt and black pepper
  Half a lemon

Pre-heat grill.
Sprinkle each fillet with dill, dot with little pieces of butter and season to taste.
Cook under a moderate heat for 4-6 minutes according to thickness of fish,
until it turns white, and flakes easily.
Squeeze lemon juice over fish and serve.

SPICED CHICKEN   ·   Serves 6

Ingredients:

  2 tsp garam masala
  1 tsp turmeric
  ½tsp ground coriander
  1 clove garlic, crushed
  10fl.oz/275ml natural yoghurt
  6 chicken thighs

Mix garam masala, turmeric, coriander and garlic into yoghurt.
Remove skin from chicken thighs and slash each two or three times.
Place chicken in a shallow ovenproof dish, spoon yoghurt mixture over to coat
chicken on both sides. Leave to marinade for 2-3 hours.
Place dish under the grill and cook for 20 minutes until golden brown, turning
once and brushing with yoghurt mixture.
Serve hot or cold with radishes and spring onions.

CHICKEN TIKKA   Serves 6

Ingredients:

> 10fl.oz/275ml natural yoghurt
> 1 tsp turmeric
> ½tsp chilli powder
> 1 tsp crushed cumin seeds
> 6 cardamom pods, bruised
> 2 cloves garlic
> 1 tsp coriander seeds, crushed and ground
> 1" peeled and finely grated fresh root ginger
> Finely grated rind and juice of half a lemon
> 6 boneless chicken breasts
> Salad of lettuce, cucumber, lemon juice and lemon wedges to
> serve

Blend yoghurt with spices, garlic, ginger, lemon rind and juice. Season well with salt and black pepper.

Cut chicken breasts into 1 inch/2.5cm cubes and add to yoghurt marinade. Mix gently to ensure chicken is well covered. Cover with lid or plastic film and chill for at least 3 hours or overnight.

Remove chicken from marinade and thread pieces on to short skewers. Set under a hot grill for 10–15 minutes, turning occasionally, until tender. Serve hot.

SYLVIA'S CHICKEN & VEGETABLE PASTIES   Serves 3

Ingredients:

> 10oz/275g flour
> 2oz/50g butter
> 5fl.oz/150ml water
> 3 pieces cooked chicken, chopped
> Cooked mixed vegetables
> Curry powder to taste

Sieve flour into food mixer and blend in butter until mixture resembles breadcrumbs. Slowly add water and mix to a soft dough. Place on a floured surface and roll out to about ½ inch/1.25cm thick and cut into three strips.

In a bowl, mix cooked vegetables and chopped cooked chicken together, adding curry powder to taste.

Distribute chicken mix between three strips of pastry, fold edges of pastry over (moisten slightly to seal) and pinch edges together

Place on a greased baking tray and cook in a moderate oven, 375F, 190C, Gas Mark 5 for approx. 15 minutes until pastry is cooked.

SPICY CHICKEN RING   Serves 4

Ingredients:
Filling:

>   2 tblsp olive oil
>   6oz/175g chicken breast
>   1 tsp curry powder
>   1 small onion, peeled and sliced
>   2 tsp cornflour
>   Seasoning to taste
>   1 small red pepper, de-seeded and sliced
>   5 tblsp water

Potato choux:

>   1oz/30g butter
>   5fl.oz/150ml water
>   2oz/50g wholemeal flour
>   Pinch of salt
>   1 egg
>   1 egg yolk
>   3oz/75g cold mashed potato

Remove skin from chicken and cut into ½ inch/1.25cm pieces. Heat oil, add chicken and cook for 5 minutes Remove with slotted spoon.

Add onion to pan and cook for 2 minutes Add red pepper and curry powder and cook for further 2 minutes Return chicken to pan and mix together gently. Mix cornflour to a smooth paste with 5 tablespoons water and stir into the mixture. Bring to the boil gradually stirring continuously, then remove from heat and season with salt and pepper.

To make the potato choux: Lightly oil a shallow, oven proof dish. Set oven to 425F, 220C, Gas Mark 7.

Measure butter and water into a pan and heat to melt the butter. Bring to the boil then quickly add all the flour and salt. Beat well, then remove from the heat and beat in the mashed potato. Cool slightly, then add egg and egg yolk and continue beating until mixture is thick and glossy.

Spoon around the edge of the prepared dish, then spoon chicken mixture into the middle. Bake in centre of oven for 25-30 minutes.

TURKEY SUPPER   Serves 2

Ingredients:

       1 crushed clove of garlic
       1 tblsp olive oil
       1 large diced onion
       ½tsp fenugreek
       6oz/175g shredded turkey
       Salt and pepper
       4oz/100g sliced green beans
       15fl.oz/425ml water
       6oz/175g fresh green tagliatelle

Put garlic, oil, fenugreek and onion into a pan. Cover and sauté. Increase heat and add turkey. Stir fry, mixing continuously, then reduce heat.
Add beans, water, salt and pepper, cover and simmer for 5 minutes. Stir in the tagliatelle and simmer for about 4 minutes. Serve.

LEEK AND CHICKEN RISOTTO   Serves 4

Ingredients:

       8oz/225g brown rice
       40fl.oz/1litre chicken stock
       3 leeks, shredded
       2 large red peppers, dices
       5oz/150g cooked chicken, diced

Put all the ingredients into a pan and season with salt and pepper.
Cover and simmer for 15-20 minutes until rice and vegetables are tender, add extra stock if necessary.

EASY CHICKEN & RICE   Serves 4

Ingredients:

      8oz/225g brown rice
      16fl.oz/425ml water
      ½ tsp salt
      2 tblsp butter
      1 small onion, finely chopped
      3 sticks celery
      3 tblsp fresh parsley, chopped
      3lbs/1.4kg chicken pieces

Put rice, water, salt, butter, onion, celery and parsley in a very large pan. Stir and bring to the boil.

Lightly salt chicken and lay it on top of the rice.

Lower heat to simmer; cover tightly and cook 45-60 minutes until water is absorbed and chicken is tender.

COUNTRY CHICKEN WITH POTATOES   Serves 4

Ingredients:

      8oz/225g onions, peeled and chopped
      1 bouquet garni
      2 cloves garlic, crushed
      10fl.oz/275ml chicken stock or water
      1lb/450g leeks, sliced thickly
      8oz/225g carrots
      8 skinned chicken drumsticks
      Salt
      Black pepper

Simmer onions, bouquet garni, garlic and stock or water for 5 minutes.

Add leeks, carrots and chicken drumsticks

Season well, cover and simmer for 40 minutes or until tender.

Serve with boiled potatoes

SAVOURY RICE   Serves 4-6

Ingredients:

> 2 tblsp oil
> 2 small onions
> 1lb/450g brown rice
> 1 tsp salt
> 60fl.oz/1.75litres vegetable water or stock
> Nutmeg, chives and parsley

Sauté chopped onions in oil, add washed rice, salt and vegetable water or stock. Cook on a low heat for 30-40 minutes until all water has been absorbed. Just before serving, sprinkle with nutmeg, chives and parsley.

BRAZILIAN RICE SALAD   Serves 4-6

Ingredients:

> 4oz/100g long grain brown rice
> 1oz/30g wild rice
> Olive oil
> 2 carrots, cut matchsticks size
> 1 red pepper, diced
> 1 onion, chopped
> 1 green pepper, diced

Cook each rice separately until tender, then mix together and trickle a little olive oil over the mix to make it shine. Add all other ingredients, mix well and serve.

STIR FRY RICE   Serves 4-6

Ingredients:

> 1lb/450g long grain brown rice
> 4oz/100g of bits!
> 4 tblsp olive oil
> 1 clove garlic, chopped
> ½"/1.25cm root ginger, chopped
> 1 egg, beaten
> 1 onion, chopped

Boil rice until tender.

In a dish, collect a selection of 'bits' such as bamboo shoots, broccoli, carrot, cauliflower, celery, chicken, duck, green pepper, lamb, leek, lobster, prawns, red pepper, shrimps. These can be fresh, or left overs, but they must all be chopped finely.

In a wok, or deep sided frying pan, heat 3 tablespoons olive oil and sauté garlic and ginger until just beginning to brown at the outer edge.

Reduce heat and add the beaten egg. Then, very quickly, add the cooked rice and turn it over in the egg mixture to coat the grains. Remove from heat and set aside.

Heat remaining 1 tablespoon olive oil and fry onion until soft. Add dish of 'bits'. Sauté together until cooked.

Add rice and egg mix to pan and cook everything together, mixing well to avoid sticking, until heated through.

LAMB CHOPS & BROWN RICE   Serves 4

Ingredients:

> 8oz/225g brown rice
> 20fl.oz/550ml boiling water
> 4 lean lamb chops
> 4oz/100g green pepper, chopped
> 2oz/50g onion, chopped
> ½tsp salt

Soak rice in boiling water for at least 30 minutes.

Brown lamb chops to seal and set aside.

Add green pepper, onion and salt to the rice and water. Simmer gently on top of stove for 10 minutes.

Pour rice mixture into lightly oiled baking dish. Layer lamb chops on top and cover.
Bake at 350F, 180C, Gas Mark 4 for 1 hour.

LAMB WITH CUMIN   Serves 4

Ingredients:
> 1 tblsp olive or safflower oil
> 2lb/900g lamb, cubed
> 1½ tsp ground cumin
> 1 tsp cumin seeds
> 6 cloves garlic, crushed
> Salt and black pepper

Heat the oil and brown the meat on all sides.
Add ground cumin, cumin seeds and garlic.
Stir and cook for 5 minutes, then add enough water to just cover and season to taste. Bring to boil.
Reduce heat, cover and simmer for 1 hour or until meat is tender.

TANGY LAMB   Serves 4

Ingredients:
> 2lb/900g lamb cut in 2"/5cm cubes
> 1 tblsp olive oil
> 2 cloves garlic, crushed
> ½ tsp ground cumin
> ½ tsp ground coriander
> ¼ tsp ground ginger
> ½ tsp turmeric or saffron
> Salt to taste
> 2 medium onions, thinly sliced
> Black pepper

Heat oil and cook meat over a moderate heat until browned on all sides.
Stir in garlic and spices, and season to taste with salt and black pepper.
Cook for further 5 minutes, then add half the onion and enough water to just cover meat.
Bring to boil, reduce heat, cover and simmer for 45 minutes then add the remaining onion. Simmer for another 45 minutes or until tender.

MIXED PEPPER PILAFF

Serves 6

Ingredients:

    20fl.oz/550ml home made stock
    6oz/175g long grain brown rice
    1 red pepper, cored, de-seeded and diced
    1 green pepper, cored, de-seeded and diced
    1 tsp ground coriander
    1 tsp ground cumin
    1 onion, peeled and finely chopped
    3 tblsp fresh chopped parsley

Place stock in a pan and bring to the boil. Add rice, peppers, coriander, cumin and onion. Bring back to boil, then reduce to simmer.
Cover and simmer for 25-30 minutes until all liquid is absorbed and rice is tender.
Stir in parsley and serve hot.

SPICED ROOTS

Serves 6

Ingredients:

    1lb/450g swede
    1lb/450g celeriac
    8oz/225g carrots
    1lb/450g onions
    1oz/30g butter
    2 tblsp oil
    1 tblsp coriander seeds, crushed
    ½ tsp turmeric
    1 tsp cumin seeds, crushed
    1pint/550ml water

Topping:

    6oz/175g plain wholemeal flour
    4oz/100g butter
    2oz/50g rolled oats with bran
    2oz/50g soda bread crumbs
    1 tsp ground cumin

Peel root vegetables and cut into large chunks. Peel and slice onions.
Melt butter with oil in a large pan and fry all vegetables for 5 minutes. Add coriander, cumin and turmeric and cook for 1 minute.

Season well and stir in 1pint/550ml water. Bring to boil, cover and simmer for 15 minutes. Mix flour, oats and soda bread crumbs in a bowl, rub in butter, add cumin. Transfer vegetables to a deep six pint/three litre casserole and spoon crumble over the top. Cook at 400F, 200C, Gas Mark 6 for 30 minutes until topping is browned.

COURGETTE AND CARROT STICKS   Serves 4

Ingredients:

> 8oz/225g courgettes
> 8oz/225g carrots
> 2oz/50g butter
> ½ tsp salt
> Ground black pepper

Wash courgettes and peel carrots.
Slice vegetables into matchstick-size pieces.
Boil carrots for 5 minutes until just tender, then hold them under cold running water for a few seconds and drain well.
Melt the butter in a large frying pan, add the courgettes and cook for 2 minutes
Add carrots and seasonings and continue to cook, stirring well, until courgettes are just soft.
Serve immediately

CUCUMBER & YOGHURT POT SALAD   Serves 8

Ingredients:

> 1lb/450g Natural Set Yoghurt
> ¼ tsp sea salt
> ¼ tsp black pepper
> 1 large clove garlic, crushed
> 1oz/30g fresh mint or dill
> 1 large cucumber

Mix the yoghurt, salt, pepper and crushed garlic together.
Blend in the mint or dill.
Cut cucumber into chunky cubes, blend with other ingredients and serve chilled.
This is very popular with curry dishes or it can be served on its own with a green salad.

IRISH POTATO SCONES

Ingredients:

>1lb/450g potatoes, mashed
>1 egg, beaten
>A little melted butter or oil
>Wholemeal flour

Add beaten egg and oil to mashed potatoes.

Mix in enough flour to stiffen, roll out and cut in rounds.

Bake on hot griddle or in oven until golden. Serve hot, lightly buttered, with vegetable pate.

WHOLEMEAL PASTA   Serves 4

Ingredients:

>8oz/225g wholemeal flour
>2 eggs
>4 tblsp water

Sift the flour into a mixing bowl.

Break the eggs, which should be at room temperature, into another mixing bowl and stir in the water.

Make a well in the centre of the flour and, using a metal whisk, gradually add the eggs, a little at a time.

Whisk well to make a smooth batter.

When all the flour has been mixed in, add the rest of the liquid. Make sure the dough is soft and firm enough to handle, not too sticky.

Knead the dough lightly on a floured surface and then either roll it out or push through a pasta maker to produce shapes.

Variation:

Beat 3oz/75g finely chopped, pre-cooked spinach with the eggs, add a little nutmeg and freshly ground black pepper to give delicious Wholemeal Pasta Verdi.

CREAMY DIP WITH CRUDITIES

Ingredients:

>   5fl.ozs/150ml natural yoghurt
>   Salt
>   2 tblsp grated cucumber
>   Pepper
>   1 dsrtsp mayonnaise
>   2 cloves garlic, crushed
>   a little chopped fresh mint

Mix all the ingredients together well and chill slightly.
Prepare a platter of raw vegetables, such as chopped carrots, sprigs of broccoli and cauliflower, spring onions, strips of pepper to eat with the dip. *(DON'T HAVE STRIPS OF PEPPER IF YOU ARE ARTHRITIC.)*

Another unusual way of serving this item is to take a sturdy lettuce leaf, spoon a small amount of dip on to it, and wrap it all up to make a delicious package.

EVE'S OATMEAL PANCAKES

Ingredients

>   10ozs/275g porridge oats
>   ¼ tsp of salt
>   ¼ tsp baking powder
>   ¼ tsp bicarbonate of soda
>   Dash of cinnamon
>   8fl.oz/225ml low fat plain yoghurt
>   1 egg, lightly beaten
>   1 tblsp butter

In the container of a blender or food processor, process oats until they are the consistency of flour.
Mix with the salt, baking powder, bicarbonate of soda and the cinnamon. Stir in the yoghurt and egg.
Melt a little butter in a frying pan over a medium heat. For each pancake spoon three tablespoons of batter into the frying pan.
Press mixture down in the pan to make it thinner so that it cooks throughout (about one and a half minutes) until lightly browned.

IRIS' SODA BREAD   Serves 4

Pick out a mug that holds eight fluid ounces or use an American measuring cup. I find an ordinary level tea cup just the right size.

Ingredients:

      5 cups wholemeal self raising flour
      Scant half cup rolled oats or fine oatmeal
      1½ level tsp bicarbonate soda
      1½ level tsp salt
      2-3 cups natural yoghurt

Pre-heat oven to 475F, 240C, Gas Mark 9 and put two shelves in centre of oven. Put all dry ingredients into a bowl and mix well together with your hands.
Add 2 cups yoghurt, adding the third one very slowly and stop when the dough is slack but not sloppy. It should spread a little when you put it on the baking tray.
Knead it lightly with the tips of the fingers. Divide into two, form each into a round and place on greased baking trays, marking each one into 8 segments with a sharp knife.
Brush tops with yoghurt and put in middle of oven, cook for 15 minutes then reduce heat to 400F, 200C, Gas Mark 6.
Swap the tins over on the shelves in the oven and cook for a further 15-20 minutes. Bread is done if it sounds hollow when tapped.

BLENDER MAYONNAISE

Ingredients:

      2 eggs at room temperature
      ¼ tsp sea salt
      2 tblsp lemon juice, fresh squeezed
      10fl.oz/275ml vegetable oil

Combine eggs, lemon juice and sea salt in a blender at high speed for 1 minute. Slowly add oil and store in a glass jar. Refrigerate

MICROWAVE SODA BREAD

Ingredients:

> 8ozs/225g wholemeal flour
> 1 level tsp salt
> ½ tsp bicarbonate of soda
> 2 oz/50g butter
> 8-10fl.oz/225-275ml of water

Mix all dry ingredients together, rub in the butter, add water and mix well.
Line a 7"/18cm microwave dish with cling film, pour in the bread mix and level out.
Cook on high power for about 6 minutes.

POTATO MASH CAKES

Ingredients:

> 3 cups leftover mashed potato
> Pinch of salt
> Pinch of mixed herbs (optional)
> 1 beaten egg
> A little rice flour to stiffen

Mix all ingredients together well and shape into flat cakes, about ½ inch/1.25cm thick.
Place on hot griddle, or in a pan lightly brushed with oil. Brown lightly on both sides.
Serve topped with cottage cheese and chopped chives.

SODA/YOGHURT BREAD

Ingredients:

> 1lb/450g self raising wholemeal flour
> 1 tsp baking powder
> ¼tsp bicarbonate of soda
> Pinch of salt
> 8ozs/225g plain yoghurt
> 5fl.oz/150ml of water.

Sieve dry ingredients into a bowl.

Blend water and yoghurt and stir well, then pour yoghurt and water mix into the dry ingredients and knead thoroughly.

Pat or roll into a round about 8 inches/20cm across and score into 8 segments. Place on a greased baking tray and put into the oven at 350F, 180C, Gas Mark 4 for 30 minutes

Cool on a wire tray and break apart so that pieces can be frozen individually to keep fresh.

1896 SODA CAKE   Serves 4

Ingredients:

> 1lb/450g plain wholemeal flour
> 1 tsp salt
> 1 tsp cream of tartar
> 10fl.oz/275ml live yoghurt
> 1 tsp bicarbonate of soda

Sieve the flour and salt into a bowl. Mix the bicarbonate of soda and cream of tartar with the yoghurt and add to flour.

Mix to a soft dough and turn onto a floured board and knead lightly. Roll out, on one side only, to about 1.5inch/4cm thick, without turning it over, bake on a hot griddle.

Alternatively, bake the cake in a moderate oven, 375F, 190C, Gas Mark 5 for about 40 minutes. Allow to cool before cutting.

RICH SAGE & ONION STUFFING

Ingredients:

> 2 large onions
> 10fl.oz/275ml water
> 3oz/75g fresh soda breadcrumbs
> 2 tsp finely chopped fresh or 1 tsp dried sage
> Salt and pepper
> 1 egg

Peel and chop onions and simmer in the water until tender. Drain and mix with breadcrumbs and sage.

Season with salt and pepper and bind with egg, moistening with a little onion stock if the mixture appears too dry.

Bake in the oven or use as stuffing for poultry.

VAL'S BREAD

Ingredients:
>   1lb/450g wholemeal flour
>   1 tblsp olive oil
>   2 generous tblsp yoghurt
>   1 egg
>   1 heaped tblsp baking powder
>   Water to mix

Put all the ingredients into a bowl and mix to a dough.
Tip onto a floured baking tray and cook in the middle of the oven at 425F, 220C, Gas Mark 7 for 40 minutes.
Turn out onto a wire rack upside down to release steam.

YOGHURT SCONES

Ingredients:
>   8 oz/225g wholemeal self-raising flour
>   ½ level tsp salt
>   1½ ozs/40g butter
>   4 tblsp natural yoghurt
>   4 tblsp water
>   A little beaten egg

Sift flour and salt into a bowl. Rub in butter finely.
Add yoghurt and water all at once and mix to a soft but not sticky dough with a knife.
Turn out onto a lightly floured board, and knead quickly until smooth. Roll out to about ¾ inch/2cm thickness.
Cut into about 9 or 10 rounds with a biscuit cutter, and transfer to a lightly buttered baking tray, brush tops with beaten egg.
Bake towards the top of a hot oven at 450F, 230C, Gas Mark 8 for 7-10 minutes, (or until golden brown.)
Cool on a wire rack, and serve lightly buttered or to choice.

STAGE 2 DIET & RECIPES

Congratulations, you have completed the first part of your treatment and should be feeling considerably better. It is now time to re-introduce some foods into your diet. However if eaten to excess these foods could cause a re-growth of your Candida so, for your own sake, don't over-indulge. Never introduce more than one new food a day, and always rotate the food within your diet, i.e. don't eat the same things on consecutive days.

You may now eat all of the items on stage 1 plus:

VEGETABLES	Artichoke (Globe and Jerusalem), Black Eye Beans, Brussel Sprouts, Green Beans, Peas, Soyabeans, Turnip
HERBS and SPICES	Bayleaf, Capers, Cayenne Pepper, Cinnamon, Mustard Seed
FISH	Dab, Pilchard, Sardine (Not in any form of ready-made sauce)
FRUIT	Apple, Apricot, Avocado, Banana, Black Olive, Cranberry, Currant, Green Olives, Kiwifruit, Mango, Melon, Peach, Pineapple, Tomatoes, Watermelon
GRAINS	Oatmeal

DAIRY PRODUCTS	Edam Cheese, Gouda Cheese, Goats' Milk, Goats' Cheese
NUTS	Chinese water chestnuts
MISCELLANEOUS	Sesame seed and oil, Tabasco Sauce

TOMATO SOUP WITH SWEET BASIL   Serves 4

Ingredients:

20fl.oz/550ml liquidized fresh ripe tomatoes
20fl.oz/550ml vegetable stock
1 carrot, grated
1 tblsp celery, finely chopped
1 tsp sweet basil, chopped
Salt and black pepper

Add basil, celery and carrot to tomatoes and seasoning.
Cover and simmer for 15 minutes. Add stock, bring to the boil and serve.

CHILLED YOGHURT & CUCUMBER SOUP   Serves 4

Ingredients:

2 medium cucumbers
16fl.oz/450ml natural yoghurt
2 tsp water
2 tsp mint, fresh chopped
Salt
Fresh ground black pepper
Sprigs of mint to decorate

Peel the cucumbers thinly with a potato peeler to remove skin but leave a little of the green colouring.
Chop cucumbers roughly and liquidise with the yoghurt and water until smooth.
Add fresh chopped mint and adjust seasoning to taste. Cover and chill for about 2 hours before serving.

SORREL SOUP   Serves 4

Ingredients:

>   2 onions, peeled and chopped
>   2 cloves garlic, peeled and crushed
>   2 tblsp olive oil
>   24oz/700g tomatoes, skinned and chopped
>   24oz/700g sorrel washed and finely chopped
>   35fl.oz/1 litre vegetable stock
>   Salt and pepper to taste

Place onions and garlic in a large pan with oil and cook for 5 minutes until soft and light brown.
Add tomatoes, sorrel, stock, salt and pepper.
Simmer for 15 minutes. Liquidise. Serve hot or cold.

SCANDINAVIAN SOUP   Serves 4

Ingredients:

>   2oz/50g butter
>   4oz/100g carrots, diced
>   4oz/100g cauliflower florets
>   4oz/100g potatoes, peeled and diced
>   2oz/50g peas
>   Scant 2oz/50g wholemeal flour
>   20fl.oz/550ml water
>   15fl.oz/425ml vegetable stock
>   Fresh ground pepper
>   Freshly chopped parsley

Melt the butter and sauté the vegetables until soft. Stir in the flour and cook for 1 minute.
Gradually stir in the water and stock. Add pepper to taste.
Simmer for 45 minutes. Garnish with parsley before serving.

MINESTRONE SOUP   Serves 4

Ingredients:

      4oz/100g Haricot beans (soaked overnight)
      60fl.oz/1.75litre vegetable stock or water
      3 carrots
      3 onions
      2-3 potatoes
      ½ small cabbage, thinly sliced
      1 turnip
      2 medium leeks
      Salt and pepper
      3 cloves garlic
      1 bayleaf
      1 pinch thyme
      1 pinch marjoram

Peel and slice all of the vegetables. Heat up the vegetable stock or water.
Heat a spoonful of olive oil in a large pan, and gently fry onion and garlic.
Add the hot stock (or water), drained haricot beans, bayleaf, thyme and marjoram. Boil on a moderate heat for 90-120 minutes until beans are tender.
Add sliced carrots, turnip and potatoes. After 10 minutes, add cabbage and leeks and boil for another 10 minutes.
Season to taste, then remove from heat and liquidise. Reheat and serve.

DRIED PEA SOUP   Serves 4

Ingredients:

      8oz/225g dried peas
      40fl.oz/1litre water
      2 onions
      1 carrot
      1 turnip
      Sprig of fresh mint
      Seasoning

Soak the peas overnight in the water.
Add the chopped vegetables into the saucepan with the peas, seasoning, and mint. Simmer gently for 75-90 minutes.
Liquidise or rub through a sieve until smooth. Re-heat, adding more seasoning if required.

CARROT SOUP   Serves 4

Ingredients:

> 4 large carrots
> 1 small turnip
> 2 stalks celery
> 1oz/30g butter
> 60fl.oz/1.75litre water
> 1oz/30g wholemeal flour
> Salt and black pepper
> Parsley (optional)

Peel and chop the vegetables and fry in the butter without browning. Add 40fl.oz/1litre water and simmer gently until tender.
Pass through a sieve or liquidiser and season to taste with salt and black pepper.
Return to saucepan, add remaining water and re heat, stirring continuously.
Blend the flour to a smooth paste with a little water and stir into the soup.
Bring to the boil, stirring continuously. Serve, sprinkled with chopped parsley.

BEST BARLEY SOUP   Serves 4

Ingredients:

> 2oz/50g whole barley
> 50fl.oz/1.25litre water
> 8oz/225g chopped carrots
> 4oz/100g chopped celery
> 2oz/50g chopped onions
> 1lb/450g chopped tomatoes
> 8oz/225g peas, fresh or frozen (unsweetened)
> Few sprigs of parsley

Cook barley in water for 1 hour. Add carrots, celery, onion, tomatoes and peas and cook until tender.
Liquidise and reheat.
Prior to serving sprinkle a little freshly chopped parsley onto each soup bowl.

EILEEN'S ARTICHOKE SOUP   Serves 4

Ingredients:
>   24oz/700g artichokes
>   1 large potato
>   1 large onion
>   2pints/1litre water
>   Salt
>   Black pepper

Peel and dice vegetables and put into water and bring to boil. Simmer until cooked thoroughly (about 45 minutes). Season to taste.
Leave to cool, then liquidise, and reheat. Serve.

BAKED TROUT IN GARLIC BUTTER   Serves 4

Ingredients:
>   4 trout fillets
>   Salt and pepper
>   4oz/100g butter
>   2 tsp garlic, finely chopped
>   Fresh parsley

Lay trout fillets in a greased oven dish, and season lightly with salt and black pepper.
Top each fillet with 1 oz/30g butter, cut into 3-4 thin flakes, and ½tsp finely chopped garlic.
Add plenty of fresh, chopped parsley, cover and bake in a hot oven for 10 minutes.

MACKEREL AND ONION PIE   Serves 2

Ingredients:

      1lb/450g white mackerel fillets
      Half cup finely chopped onion
      2 tblsp finely chopped parsley
      2 lbs/900g potatoes
      2 tblsp butter
      Salt to taste
      ½ cup water

Wash fillets and cut in pieces. Lay a few pieces in an oiled pie dish, sprinkle with chopped onion and parsley, and salt lightly. Continue in layers until fish, onion and parsley have all been used.

Boil potatoes and then mash them, beat in the butter, season to taste and make into a soft paste with the water.

Spread potato mash over fish layers and ripple with the back of a fork, dot with a little extra butter and bake for about 20 minutes at 375F, 190C, Gas Mark 5.

JAMBALAYA   Serves 4-6

Ingredients:

      2 stalks of celery
      1 large onion
      2 tblsp cooking oil
      1-2 tsp chilli powder
      12ozs/350g long grain brown rice
      2 bay leaves
      14oz/450g canned, chopped tomatoes.
      35fl.oz/1 litre chicken stock
      1 red pepper
      1 green pepper
      1lb/450g cooking prawns (defrosted)

Chop the celery and onion and cook in the oil until soft. Add chilli powder and rice and cook for 2 to 3 minutes. Add bay leaves, tomatoes and most of the stock. Cover and simmer for 5 minutes.

Remove core and seeds from the peppers, slice and add them to the pan. Continue cooking gently for a further 10-15 minutes, until the rice is cooked, adding more stock as necessary.

Rinse the prawns in cold water, drain, then add to the rice mixture. Heat through gently.

Add salt and pepper to taste. Garnish and serve with garlic bread and a crisp green salad.

FISH HOTPOT   Serves 4

Ingredients:

    12oz/350g white fish
    1½lbs/675g potatoes
    2 small onions
    8oz/225g tomatoes
    Salt and black pepper
    Bouquet garni
    15fl.oz/425ml water
    1oz/30g butter

Cut fish into neat pieces. Peel and slice potatoes, onions and tomatoes and arrange in layers, with the fish, in a deep casserole, sprinkling each layer with salt and pepper. Add bouquet garni, half cover with water and finish with a layer of potato on top.

Cover and cook in a very moderate, 350F, 180C, Gas Mark 4 for about 45 minutes

Remove lid, dot top with butter and cook for a further 15 minutes. Remove bouquet garni before serving.

MARINATED CHICKEN   Serves 4

Ingredients:

    2 cloves garlic, crushed
    1 tsp ground cumin
    1"/2.5cm fresh root ginger, grated
    ½tsp chilli powder
    6oz/175g strained natural yoghurt
    ¼tsp turmeric
    3 large chicken breasts, skinned and boned.

Mix garlic, spices and ginger. Stir into yoghurt.

Chop chicken in ½inch/1.25cm cubes and stir in yoghurt mixture. Place in ovenproof dish, cover and chill for 4-6 hours or overnight.

Preheat oven to 350F, 180C, Gas Mark 4. Stir mixture and place in the bottom of the oven. Cook slowly for 40 minutes and serve hot. This can also be left to go completely cold and served with a side salad.

BASILY CHICKEN   Serves 4

Ingredients:
> 4 chicken breasts
> 1 tomato, sliced into 8
> A little dried basil
> Dried garlic granules to taste
> 10fl.oz/275ml pint chicken stock
> Ground black pepper

Using a sharp knife, carefully make slits in each chicken breast to form a pocket. Sprinkle sliced tomato with dried basil and garlic granules.
Place tomatoes in chicken pockets and arrange chicken in an ovenproof dish with chicken stock. Sprinkle with ground black pepper.
Cover and cook in a moderate oven, 375F, 190C, Gas Mark 5 for 30-40 minutes or until tender.

CHICKEN IN YOGHURT SAUCE   Serves 4

Ingredients:
> 10oz/275ml natural set yoghurt
> 1 tsp chilli powder
> 1oz/30g fresh coriander
> ½tsp ground cumin
> 1oz/30g fresh ginger
> 1 clove of garlic, crushed
> 4 x 10oz/275g chicken breasts
> Fresh parsley

Blend yoghurt, chilli powder, coriander, cumin, ginger and garlic and leave in a bowel overnight. Pierce chicken pieces all over with a fork and pour on half of the yoghurt mix. Allow to stand for 2 hours.
Place the marinade and the chicken into a roasting tin, cover and cook for 40 mins at 400F, 200C, Gas Mark 6.
Remove from oven, place roasting tin on the top of the gas or electric ring, add the remaining yoghurt mix, bring to the boil, then reduce heat slightly. Serve very hot with sprigs of fresh parsley to decorate.

RICE STUFFED PEPPERS   Serves 4

Ingredients:

2 large green peppers
3oz/75g brown rice
1–2oz/30–50g butter
1 large onion
½ clove garlic
2 large tomatoes, sliced
Salt and black pepper

Cut green peppers into halves across the middle. Remove cores and seeds. Put peppers into boiling, salted water and cook for 5 minutes only.
Boil rice until tender, (about 15 minutes).
Drain peppers and rice well.
Heat butter and fry onion, garlic and sliced tomatoes. Fry until soft. Mix with rice and season well.
Pile into the 4 halves of peppers and put into a moderate oven, 375F, 190C, Gas Mark 5 and bake for 25 minutes.

COLOURFUL RICE & VEGETABLES   Serves 4

Ingredients:

1 mug frozen peas, without added sugar
1 mug frozen french beans
1 mug long grain rice
½ chicken stock cube, yeast free
2 mugs boiling water or home made chicken stock

Put all the ingredients in an ovenproof dish. Stir to mix well.
Cover with foil and bake at 350F, 180C, Gas Mark 4 for 50 minutes.

This makes an excellent main meal for two, or can be used for four people if served with a main course such as fish.

PAELLA   Serves 4

Ingredients:
>   4 tblsp olive oil
>   10oz/275g long grain brown rice
>   1 large onion, peeled and sliced
>   2 large cloves of garlic, crushed
>   ½ packet saffron
>   25fl.oz/700ml vegetable stock or water
>   Freshly ground black pepper
>   4oz/100g peas, without added sugar
>   1 red pepper, de-seeded and sliced
>   Chopped parsley

Heat oil in a large, deep pan. Add rice and onion, stirring until rice turns opaque.

Add garlic, saffron, stock and pepper. Mix well and bring to boil. Mix again, ensuring saffron colouring is evenly distributed.

Add sliced red pepper and peas, bring back to the boil, cover and simmer gently for 45 minutes. Serve, sprinkled with chopped parsley.

ORIENTAL RICE   Serves 4

Ingredients:
>   2 onions
>   4 tblsp olive oil
>   8oz/225g long grain brown rice
>   30fl.oz/850ml chicken stock (hot)
>   8oz/225g mixed cooked vegetables
>   4oz/100g prawns

Chop onions very finely and fry with the rice in the oil until just brown, stirring frequently to prevent the rice sticking.

Add the hot stock to the rice, cover and simmer for 10 minutes.

Add the rest of the ingredients and simmer for a further 10 minutes or until the rice has absorbed all of the liquid. Serve hot.

RICE & CHEESE   Serves 2

Ingredients:

> 1 egg
> 1 cup goats' milk
> ½ cup grated cheese
> Pinch of salt
> 1 small onion, chopped finely
> 2 cups cooked brown rice
> ½ tblsp oil

Beat egg lightly, then beat in the milk.
Add the rest of the ingredients, except the oil, and mix thoroughly.
Brush a casserole dish with the oil. Turn mixture into it and bake in a moderate
oven, 350F, 180C Gas Mark 4 until set.

COUNTRY BEANS   Serves 6

Ingredients:

> 1lb/450g mixed dried beans
> 30fl.oz/850ml boiling water
> 1lb/450g onions
> 2 tblsp oil
> 2 cloves garlic crushed
> 2 tsp ground cumin
> ½tsp chilli powder
> 2 tsp ground coriander
> 14oz/400g can tomatoes
> 2 tblsp tomato purée
> 20fl.oz/550ml vegetable stock

Topping:

> 1oz/30g soda bread crumbs
> ½tsp dried crushed chillies
> a little butter

Cover beans with boiling water and soak for 1 hour. Drain and put in a large
pan. Cover with cold water, bring to the boil and boil rapidly for 10 minutes.
Cover and simmer for about 50 minutes or until they are tender.
Peel and slice onions. Fry in the oil until soft. Stir in garlic, ground cumin, chilli
powder and coriander. Cook for 1 minute.

Stir in tomatoes, tomato purée, drained beans, and stock. Season. Bring to the boil. Transfer to a deep 4pint/2 litre casserole.

Sprinkle breadcrumbs and crushed chillies over. Dot with butter. Cook at 350F, 180C, Gas Mark 4 for 1 hour until crumbs are golden.

BLACK EYE BEANS IN RED SAUCE`   Serves 2

Ingredients:

> 10oz/275g black eye beans
> 4fl.oz/100ml olive oil
> ½tsp cayenne pepper
> ½tblsp paprika
> Crispy lettuce

Soak the beans overnight and cook until soft, remembering to keep the cooking liquor.

Heat the olive oil in a deep pan. Add cayenne pepper, stir well to release aroma. Add paprika, stir well and add cooked beans and about 5fl.oz/150ml of the bean liquor. Stir again and simmer until beans are very hot.

Serve on a bed of crispy lettuce.

SAVOURY BEAN FRITTERS   Serves 4

Ingredients:

> 12oz/350g dried haricot beans
> 1 tsp dried ginger
> 2 tblsp olive oil
> 1 onion
> 1 clove garlic, crushed
> 1 tsp salt
> Pinch chilli powder
> ¼tsp black pepper

Soak beans overnight in cold water to cover. Bring to boil in same water and add ginger. Cook, covered, over low heat for 2 hours or until very tender. When beans are tender you should have no water left.

Gently mash beans with a potato masher so that they are fully crushed and smooth.

Heat the oil in a large heavy pan. Add the finely chopped onion and garlic and cook for 3 minutes.

Add mashed beans, salt, chilli powder and pepper. Heat for 5-10 minutes, stirring, until thoroughly hot. Mixture should be dry; add more seasoning if required.

Form into flat cakes when cool. Heat enough oil in frying pan to give ½ inch/ 1.25cm depth. Fry bean cakes until brown. Drain on absorbent paper.

LAMB IN ROSEMARY & TOMATO SAUCE   Serves 6

Ingredients:

> 6 thick cut lamb steaks or chops
> 1 sprig of fresh rosemary
> 4 tblsp olive oil
> 2lb/900g ripe tomatoes
> 6 spring onions
> 1 clove garlic, crushed

Wipe lamb, wash and dry rosemary sprigs. Put lamb, rosemary and 2 tablespoons oil in a dish and marinate for at least 4 hours, preferably overnight.

Skin tomatoes by plunging them into boiling water for 30 seconds, then into cold water. Peel away skins, chop tomatoes roughly.

Thinly slice spring onions, add to tomatoes with garlic and remaining oil. Use a potato masher to crush tomatoes without making sauce completely smooth. Season and chill thoroughly.

Lift lamb out of oil and cook on the barbecue for 10 minutes. (Put a few sprigs of fresh rosemary in among the coals, if liked.) Turn steaks, cook for a further 5 minutes or until cooked to personal preference.

Pour the chilled tomato sauce over the hot lamb steaks and serve with a side salad.

LAMB KOFTAS   Serves 4

Ingredients:

> 8oz/225g lean minced lamb
> ½ onion, grated
> 2 tsp tomato purée
> 2 tsp freshly chopped mint
> 1 tsp salt
> 1 tsp ground cumin
> 3oz/75gm fresh sodabread crumbs
> 1 very small egg, beaten
> 8 baby onions, peeled
> 1 red pepper, de-seeded and cut into 1"/2.5cm squares

Mix together minced lamb, grated onion, tomato purée, freshly chopped mint, salt and ground cumin. Add fresh sodabread crumbs and beaten egg, mix with hands and shape into 12 meatballs.

Thread onto each skewer, 3 meatballs, 2 baby onions and squares of red pepper. Mould meatballs around skewers.

Chill for 2 hours, brush with oil, place under a pre heated grill for 15-20 minutes, turning and brushing with oil.

LAMB CHOP CASSEROLE   Serves 4

Ingredients:

> 10oz/275g package frozen green beans
> 2 large onions, sliced
> 4 potatoes, peeled and sliced
> 4 lean lamb chops
> Salt to taste

Layer beans, onions and potatoes in a lightly oiled casserole or baking tin. Sprinkle lightly with salt.

Place lamb chops on top, cover and bake at 375F, 190C, Gas Mark 5 for 45 minutes.

Remove cover, or foil, and bake for an additional 15 minutes until chops are tender and brown.

LAMB CHOPS WITH WATERCRESS SAUCE   Serves 6

Ingredients:

> 1 chopped onion
> 1oz/30g butter
> 1 bunch watercress, chopped
> 2 potatoes, diced
> 15fl.oz/425ml chicken stock
> 3 tblsp yoghurt
> 6 loin chops of lamb
> Black pepper
> 1 tsp dried rosemary

Sauté the onion in the butter, add watercress and cook for 5 minutes. Add diced potatoes and season well.

Pour in chicken stock and simmer gently for 15 minutes until potato is soft.

Blend or rub through a sieve.

Return to pan, heat gently and stir in the yoghurt.

While sauce is simmering, sprinkle the chops with plenty of ground black pepper and a little rosemary.

Grill for 10-15 minutes on both sides and put onto serving plates.

Pour sauce over chops and serve with new potatoes and a green vegetable.

LAMB STIR FRY   Serves 4

Ingredients:

>   1lb/450g thin strips lamb leg steaks
>   1 tblsp oil
>   1 carrot
>   1 courgette
>   ½ red pepper
>   ½ yellow pepper
>   Salt and pepper
>   6oz/175g beansprouts

Slice all vegetables into thin strips

Heat oil in a frying pan or wok. When very hot add the lamb and brown quickly. Add carrot and stir-fry, stirring continuously for 2 minutes.

Add courgette and peppers and stir-fry for about 3 minutes.

Add beansprouts and fry for 2 minutes, add seasoning to taste, and serve over boiled brown rice.

GOLDEN VEGETABLE PIE   Serves 6

Ingredients:

>   1 large onion, sliced
>   2 tblsp olive oil
>   1 large turnip, diced
>   3 carrots, sliced
>   1 large parsnip, diced
>   1 small swede, diced
>   2 cloves garlic, crushed
>   2 tsp turmeric
>   2 tsp crushed coriander seeds
>   1 tsp cumin seeds
>   25fl.oz/700ml vegetable stock

Sesame Pastry:
>   3 tblsp sesame seeds
>   4oz/100g butter
>   8oz/225g self raising wholemeal flour

Heat oil in a large saucepan and fry all vegetables for 5 minutes.
Add garlic, turmeric and crushed seeds and cook for 1 minute.
Pour in stock, season, cover and cook for 15 minutes until vegetables are tender.
Spoon into a 2 pint/1 litre pie dish and cool.
Place sesame seeds in a frying pan and heat gently until toasted.
Place flour in a large bowl with a pinch of salt. Rub the butter into the flour,
stir in sesame seeds. Add 8-10 tablespoons water and mix to soft dough.
Knead lightly on a floured surface and roll out. Brush the dish edge with water
and cover filling. Brush top of pie with beaten egg and cook at 400F, 200C,
Gas Mark 6 for 45 minutes.

STIR FRY VEGETABLE SCRAMBLE   Serves 1

Ingredients:
>   2 tblsp olive oil or butter
>   2 tblsp chopped onion
>   2 tblsp chopped green pepper
>   4oz/100g chopped tomato
>   8oz/225g cooked vegetables
>   2 eggs

Heat a wok or frying-pan and add oil, onions and green peppers, stir until
tender.
Add tomatoes and other vegetables. Bring to boil, stirring constantly.
Add lightly beaten eggs and cook, stirring gently. Serve immediately.

VEGETABLE RISOTTO   Serves 4

Ingredients:

        4oz/100g chopped onion
        2 tsp butter
        1 tsp olive oil
        8oz/225g long grain brown rice
        30fl.oz/850ml boiling water
        1 heaped tsp dried tarragon
        ¼tsp black pepper
        Good pinch of ground nutmeg
        ¼tsp salt
        1lb/450g frozen mixed vegetables (without added sugar)

Gently fry chopped onion in butter and olive oil until soft. Stir in rice.
Add boiling water, return to boil and simmer gently for 15 minutes. Stir in
tarragon, ground black pepper, nutmeg, salt and frozen mixed vegetables.
Cover and continue to cook until the rice and vegetables are tender and all the
liquid has been absorbed. Serve immediately.

SPRING VEGETABLE BRAISE   Serves 4

Ingredients:

        1 onion, peeled and chopped
        4 tblsp olive oil
        1lb/450g young carrots
        8oz/225g young turnips
        8oz/225g mangetout
        8oz/225g quartered cauliflower florets
        5fl.oz/150ml water
        Freshly ground black pepper
        2-3 tblsp fresh chopped parsley

Sauté onion in olive oil for 10 minutes, until soft. Scrape or scrub, carrots and
turnips. Cut in quarters. Wash, top and tail mange tout.
Add all chopped vegetables to the sautéed onion and mix gently so that they
are all covered in oil. Cook for about 2 minutes, then add water.
Cover and simmer gently for 7-8 minutes until all vegetables are tender. Season,
sprinkle with chopped parsley and black pepper. Serve.

GARLIC SAUTÉED POTATOES   Serves 4

Ingredients:
> 1–2lb/450–900g scrubbed potatoes
> 4 tblsp olive oil
> 2 cloves garlic, peeled and chopped
> 1 onion, thinly sliced
> 1 tblsp sesame seeds
> Fresh chopped parsley to garnish

Parboil potatoes for 5 minutes and slice.
Fry garlic and onion in oil for 3 minutes. Add sliced potatoes and fry, turning frequently until browned.
Add sesame seeds and cook for 2 minutes. Serve hot, topped with parsley.

MEDITERRANEAN POTATOES   Serves 8

Ingredients:
> 1 bulb garlic cloves
> 2 bouquet garni
> 20fl.oz/550ml water
> 12 medium potatoes sliced thickly
> 8 large tomatoes, sliced thickly
> Salt, pepper

Put garlic, bouquet garni and water in a pan. Simmer for 30 minutes Cool, then remove bouquet garni.
Peel garlic and pound with water from pan until smooth.
Spoon half the garlic residue into ovenproof dish. Arrange potatoes and tomatoes in layers on top and season well with salt and pepper. Spoon over remaining garlic residue.
Cover with foil and cook in a moderate oven, 350F, 180C, Gas Mark 4 for 60–75 minutes or until potatoes are tender. Garnish with parsley.

SPICY STUFFED CABBAGE   Serves 4

Ingredients:

> 24oz/700g minced lamb
> 1 onion, peeled and chopped
> 2 cloves garlic, crushed
> 1 tsp ground allspice
> ½tsp ground cinnamon
> 14oz/400g can tomatoes
> 5fl.oz/150ml water
> Salt and pepper
> Generous 2lb/1kg green cabbage

Dry fry mince in a saucepan, stirring, until evenly browned. Add onion and garlic to pan and fry until soft. Stir in allspice, cinnamon, tomatoes, water and seasoning and cook for 20 minutes.

Trim off any damaged outer cabbage leaves. Hollow out the centre in small sections with a grapefruit knife, leaving three outer layers of leaves only.

Spoon mince mixture into centre of cabbage and in between leaves. Place stuffed cabbage in steamer, cover and steam for 20 minutes until tender but still bright green. To serve, cut cabbage into wedges.

RATATOUILLE   Serves 4

Ingredients:

> 1 large aubergine, chopped
> 3 medium onions, peeled and sliced
> 2 cloves garlic, crushed
> 2 tblsp olive oil
> 2 courgettes, sliced
> 1 large yellow pepper
> 1 large red pepper
> 2x14oz/400g cans tomatoes
> 1 tblsp fresh chopped mixed herbs
> 5fl.oz/150ml hot chicken stock
> Salt and pepper
> Chopped parsley to garnish

Place chopped aubergine on a board or plate, and sprinkle with salt. Leave for 1 hour, then rinse and pat dry.

In a large deep frying pan, fry onions and garlic in olive oil for 5 minutes until soft and opaque. Add aubergine and courgettes and fry for a further 3-4 minutes, stirring occasionally.

Add squares of red and yellow peppers and cook for a further 2 minutes

Drain almost all of the liquid from the tomatoes and add them to the pan. (Save the liquid for another recipe!) Gently stir in the chopped mixed herbs, taking care not to break the tomatoes. Cook for another 2-3 minutes.

Stir in hot chicken stock, add salt and pepper to taste and simmer for 5-10 minutes until all vegetables are just tender. Sprinkle over a little chopped parsley to garnish.

This can be served hot or cold. To freeze: Pack into handy sized polythene boxes and freeze. Use within 6 months.

ITALIAN SALAD   Serves 4

Ingredients:

    1 aubergine, cut in ½"/1.25cm slices
    1 red pepper
    1 green pepper
    2 tomatoes
    1 onion
    1 clove garlic
    4 tblsp olive oil
    1 courgette, cut in ½"/1.25cm slices
    Salt and pepper
    8oz/225g wholemeal pasta spirals

Sprinkle aubergine with salt and leave for 30 minutes

Core and de-seed peppers. Cut in ½"/1.25cm slices. Skin and roughly chop tomatoes. Peel and chop onion and garlic.

Heat 3 tablespoons olive oil in pan, and fry onion gently until transparent but not brown.

Rinse salt from aubergine and pat dry with absorbent paper. Chop roughly.

Add aubergine, courgette, peppers, tomatoes and garlic to onion and fry gently for 20 minutes. Season with salt and pepper and allow to cool.

Meanwhile, cook pasta spirals in boiling salted water for 10 minutes, or until tender but still firm. Rinse in cold water and drain well. Toss in remaining olive oil, add vegetables and toss well together.

COURGETTES SAUTÉED WITH MARJORAM   Serves 4

Ingredients:

>   6 medium courgettes
>   1 large onion
>   1 clove garlic, chopped
>   1 tsp fresh marjoram, chopped
>   3 tblsp olive oil
>   8 tblsp vegetable stock
>   Salt and pepper
>   2 medium tomatoes, peeled and chopped

Chop courgettes, onion, garlic and marjoram. Peel and chop tomatoes.
Heat oil in a large frying pan. Cook onion and garlic together until tender. Add courgettes, marjoram and stock and season well.
Cover and simmer for 8-10 minutes. Add tomatoes and cook for a further 2 minutes. Serve at once

APPLE & POTATO MASH   Serves 4

Ingredients:

>   1lb/450g potatoes
>   2 medium onions
>   1 tblsp olive oil
>   8oz/225g cooking apples
>   ¼tsp black pepper
>   ¼tsp salt
>   ¼tsp ground nutmeg
>   1oz/30g butter

Boil potatoes in lightly salted water until soft.
Peel and finely chop onion. Heat oil, add onion and cook until soft and opaque.
Peel, core and slice apple, add to pan with onions, cover and simmer for 10 minutes until apples turn to pulp. Stir in salt, pepper and nutmeg.
Strain cooked potatoes and mash with butter. Add apple and onion mixture, combine with a fork. Serve immediately.

BANANA OAT CAKE

Ingredients:

      1lb/450g oat flour
      ¼tsp salt
      2 tsp baking powder
      2 eggs
      3 tblsp cold water
      2 tblsp unrefined vegetable oil
      4oz/100g mashed banana

Mix all dry ingredients together.

Beat eggs. Add water, oil and mashed banana to eggs. Blend egg mixture with dry ingredients.

Put into a lightly greased baking tin. Cook at 350°F, 180°C, Gas Mark 4 for 25-30 minutes.

RICE MUFFINS   Makes 12

Ingredients:

      1½ cups rice flour
      ½tsp salt
      2 tsp baking powder
      ¼tsp baking soda
      4 tblsp unrefined vegetable oil
      1 cup water
      3 tblsp apricot, puréed, (NO added sugar)

Lightly grease muffin or bun tins, and preheat oven to 350F, 180C, Gas Mark 4. Mix all ingredients together well and divide equally between 12 tins. Bake for 15-20 minutes.

RICE AND ROSEMARY STUFFING

Ingredients:

> 2 cups brown rice, cooked
> 2 tblsp olive oil
> ½ cup finely chopped onion
> ⅛tsp salt
> ½ cup finely chopped carrot
> ⅛tsp rosemary

Put rice in bowl, stir with a fork to separate grains.
Add all other ingredients and mix well. Use to stuff poultry.

OAT BISCUITS   Makes approx. 24

Ingredients:

> 6oz/175g butter
> 1 beaten free range egg
> 4oz/100g apple peeled and grated
> 10oz/275g wholemeal self-raising flour
> 2oz/50g breakfast oats

Set oven to 375F, 190C, Gas Mark 5.
Beat butter until soft, add egg, grated apple and flour and mix well until blended
to a fairly dry dough. Weigh dough out into ½ ounce/15g pieces and roll into
the size of a plum, then roll in the oats until well covered.
Place dough balls on greased trays, flatten with a pallet knife and bake for 20–
25 minutes until golden brown.

APPLE SCONES   Makes 8-10

Ingredients:

        8oz/225g wholemeal self raising flour
        1 level tsp baking powder
        2oz/50g butter
        3oz/75g apple, peeled and grated
        2 dsrtsp live yoghurt
        A little water to mix

Rub butter into flour and baking powder. Mix in the apple.
Mix in yoghurt, (it's handy to 'cut in' with the blade of a knife). Combine with
a little water to make into a soft dough.
Roll out to about three-quarters of 1"/2cm thick and cut into 8 or 10 scones.
Bake at 450°F, 230°C, Gas Mark 8 for about 10 minutes or until golden brown.
Serve warm, lightly buttered.

NOTE: Substitute the apple with banana or pear for a change.

STAGE 3 DIET & RECIPES

Well done! You have progressed this far and should, by now, be a completely different person to the one who started treatment. However, you must still exercise caution. Add the following foods to your stage 1 and stage 2 lists. As before, never introduce more than 1 new item a day and rotate all your food as much as possible.

VEGETABLES   Aduki Beans, Chickpeas, Carob, Kidney Beans, Lentils, Lima Beans, Spinach, Split Peas, Mung Beans, Tofu

FISH   Haddock, Hake, Halibut

FRUITS   Blackberry, Boysenberry, Blueberry, Cherry, Crab-apple, Gooseberry, Kumquat, Lemon, Lime, Peach, Pineapple, Plum, Prune, Satsuma, Strawberry

GRAINS   Bran, Buckwheat, Millet, Oats

DAIRY PRODUCE
               Cheddar Cheese, Cheshire Cheese, Parmesan

NUTS   Almond, Cashew, Chestnuts, Filbert, Peanut, Pecan, Hazelnut

MISCELLANEOUS
               Peanut Oil, Soya Flour, Soya Milk, Soya Oil

PEA SOUP   Serves 1

Ingredients

 1oz/30g split peas, yellow or green
 1 bay leaf
 4 black peppercorns
 1 onion diced
 1 leek diced
 1 carrot diced
 10fl.oz/275ml water

Soak the peas overnight.
Boil peas with bay leaf and peppercorns for 20 minutes.
Prepare remaining vegetables and place them in a saucepan with a lid and small amount of water to cook in their own steam on top of the stove for about 10 minutes. Alternatively, cook on high in the microwave for 5 minutes. Stir frequently.
Add peas and water and simmer for approx. 30 minutes. Season to taste and serve.

TOMATO & LENTIL SOUP   Serves 4

Ingredients:

 2oz/50g lentils
 30fl.oz/850ml chicken or vegetable stock
 12oz/350g tomatoes
 Salt and ground black pepper
 Knob of butter
 Bouquet garni

Soak lentils overnight in the stock. Add tomatoes, salt and pepper. Simmer for 60-75 minutes until tender.
Sieve or liquidise and beat well with a wooden spoon. Reheat with butter and herbs for 10-15 minutes.
Remove bouquet garni before serving.

PRAWN CHOWDER   Serves 6

Ingredients:

> 1lb/450g Finnan haddock
> 30fl.oz/850ml water
> ½ lemon, sliced
> 1lb/450g potatoes, peeled
> 1 bunch spring onions
> 1oz/30g butter
> 4oz/100g prawns
> Pinch grated nutmeg

Place haddock in a saucepan with water, and lemon slices. Bring to boil and simmer gently for 5 minutes.
Cut potatoes into small dice and chop spring onions.
Lift out fish with a fish slice. Strain liquid and reserve. Wipe saucepan dry and melt butter.
Add potatoes and spring onions, fry for 3 minutes. Return water to pan and simmer for 5 minutes.
Remove bones and skin from haddock and flake with fork. Add to pan with prawns, nutmeg and seasoning.
Simmer for 5 minutes Serve.

RUNNER BEAN SOUP   Serves 3

Ingredients:

> 20fl.oz/550ml water
> Salt to taste
> 1 cup chopped runner beans
> 1 large raw potato, grated
> 15fl.oz/425ml goats' milk or soya milk

Bring water and salt to boil. Drop in runner beans.
Add the raw, grated potato and boil till beans are tender. Remove and cool.
Liquidise and strain off fibres, or sieve.
Add milk, re-heat until just short of boiling and serve.

SCOTCH BROTH   Serves 4

Ingredients:

      12-16oz/350-450g mutton
      3pt/1.5litre cold water or vegetable stock
      ½ turnip
      ½ celery stalk
      ½ onion
      ½ carrot
      1 tsp fine chopped parsley
      1 tblsp millet
      salt to taste

Cut meat in very small pieces, carefully removing any fragments of bone. Put into a pan with water or stock and simmer gently for 2½ hours.

Dice prepared vegetables and add to broth, with millet. Continue simmering for about 30 minutes until millet is very tender. Strain and return broth to pan. Cut meat into very small pieces, carefully removing any fragments of bone and return all of these to the broth.

Re-heat, and season to taste. Before serving sprinkle with chopped parsley.

KEDGEREE   Serves 4

Ingredients:

      8oz/225g haddock
      Knob of butter
      12oz/350g brown rice
      3 onions
      Olive oil
      3 sliced hard-boiled eggs
      Salt and black pepper
      Pinch of curry powder

Put haddock in a baking tin with a little water and cover with a piece of lightly buttered paper. Bake in a moderate oven, 350F, 180C, Gas Mark 4 for 20 minutes until the fish comes off the skin easily.

Drain, remove any skin and bone and flake. Keep warm.

Boil rice until soft and fluffy in individual grains. Keep warm.

Slice onions, chop roughly and fry in a little olive oil over a moderate heat until soft and golden. Sprinkle with salt, pepper and curry powder.

Mix fish, eggs and onions into the rice. Stir gently with a fork and serve.

HADDOCK JULIENNE   Serves 4

Ingredients:

      24oz/700g fresh haddock fillet
      1 carrot, cut into fine strips
      ½ leek, trimmed and shredded
      5fl.oz/150ml tomato juice
      1 lemon, finely grated rind only
      1 tsp fresh dill, chopped
      8 fresh mint sprigs
      Salt and ground black pepper

Cut fish into 4 neat pieces and place each one on a square of cooking foil.
Divide the carrot and leek into 4 and scatter over the fish. Pour tomato juice over the fish.
Scatter lemon rind and dill over the top and add a mint sprig to each parcel. Season to taste.
Bring the foil up round each piece of fish and pleat the edges together on top to make neat parcels.
Place on a baking sheet and bake at 375F, 190C, Gas Mark 5 for 20 minutes
Just before serving, neatly unfold the foil, re move the mint sprigs and replace with fresh ones.

LEMON BUTTERMINT TROUT   Serves 2

Ingredients:

      2 trout fillets
      Salt and black pepper
      2oz/50g butter
      Small lemon
      2 tblsps chopped fresh mint

Season trout fillets lightly with salt and black pepper.
Melt 1oz/30g of the butter in a non-stick pan, sauté the trout gently for 3-4 minutes each side.
Add a further 1oz/30g butter, the juice and grated rind of a small lemon, and the fresh mint.
Heat gently through, season to taste and serve immediately.

BAKED STUFFED HERRINGS   Serves 4

Ingredients:

> 1 shallot or small onion
> 4 sprigs parsley
> 1 cup brown rice, cooked
> 1 tblsp olive oil.
> ¼tsp salt
> 1 egg, well beaten
> 4 large herrings

Chop onion and parsley very finely. Mix with rice, oil and salt. Bind together with an egg.

Split herrings, remove backbone and as many small bones as possible. Divide mixture equally between herrings. Fold over and secure with strong cotton. Place in an oiled casserole, cover and bake at 375F, 190C, Gas Mark 5 for 10 minutes.

Remove covering and bake for a further 10 minutes.

LEMON MARINADED SARDINES   Serves 4

Ingredients:

> 6 tblsp lemon juice
> ½tsp paprika
> 2 tblsp olive oil
> 2 bay leaves
> ½tsp salt
> Black pepper to taste
> 1 onion
> 1 garlic clove, crushed
> 1lb/450g sardines
> 1 lemon to garnish

Mix the lemon juice, paprika, olive oil, bay leaves, salt and pepper.

Chop the onion very finely. Crush the garlic. Add onion and garlic to the lemon mixture.

Arrange the sardines in a dish, pour the marinade over and cover with Clingfilm and refrigerate for 24 hours, turning occasionally.

Remove Clingfilm, barbecue or grill under medium heat until skin begins to brown. Serve with lemon wedges.

LEMONY SKATE WITH CAPERS   Serves 4

Ingredients:

        2 wings of skate, approx 2lbs/900g
        1 lemon
        2 tsp chopped fresh tarragon
        Salt and pepper
        ½ cucumber
        ½ bunch radishes
        1 tsp capers
        3 tblsp oil
        Sprig of fresh tarragon

Cut each skate wing in half and cut ½ inch/1.25cm from frilly outer edge with scissors.

Peel the rind from lemon using a vegetable peeler, squeeze lemon juice and reserve.

Arrange skate overlapping in the steamer so that the thickest part of each piece is on the base. Sprinkle with lemon rind, tarragon and seasoning. Cover and steam for 7 minutes.

Slice cucumber and quarter radishes.

Re-arrange skate so that pieces from middle are now on top or bottom. Arrange vegetables on top. Cook for 3 minutes or until fish is tender.

Chop capers. Mix lemon juice, oil and seasoning.

Place skate on serving plates, sprinkle with capers. Toss vegetables in lemon mix, serve with skate, garnish with tarragon

JAMAICAN CHICKEN & LENTILS   Serves 4

Ingredients:

        4oz/100g lentils
        20fl.oz/550ml water
        8oz/225g brown rice
        2 grated carrots
        1 onion, chopped
        1 clove garlic, crushed
        1 knob butter
        Salt and pepper to taste
        8oz/225g cooked chicken
        Mustard and cress

Wash lentils and simmer in the water for 30 minutes until soft.
Put rice in a large saucepan, cover with cold water and bring slowly to the boil.
Reduce the heat and simmer until tender, adding a little more water if necessary.
Drain both the lentils and rice.
Mix all of the ingredients together, except the chicken and cook gently for 15 minutes.
Add the chicken, mix well and cook for a further 5-10 minutes. Serve, garnished with mustard and cress.

LEMON CHICKEN   Serves 4

Ingredients:

> 4 chicken breasts boned and skinned
> 1 large carrot
> 2 sticks celery
> 20fl.oz/550ml chicken stock
> 1 tsp butter
> 2 tsp flour
> Salt and black pepper
> ½ lemon, juice and rind
> 3 spring onions, thinly sliced

Place chicken in a single layer on the base of a large saucepan, add vegetables, cut into julienne strips.
Add chicken stock and lemon juice, cover and bring to boil. Reduce heat to low and cook for a further 20 minutes. Turn off heat and leave for a further 10 minutes.
Remove chicken and vegetables, and keep hot.
Cream together butter and flour. Gradually add in stock and whisk over a medium heat until thickened. Simmer for 2 minutes, add salt and pepper if required.
Divide vegetables between each plate, cut each chicken breast into thick slices and lay on plate, pour over sauce. Garnish with lemon rind and spring onion.
Serve with vegetables or side salad.

LENTIL LOAF   Serves 4

Ingredients:

      8oz/225g lentils
      2oz/50g butter
      2 chopped onions
      2 large tomatoes, skinned
      1 small apple, peeled, cored and chopped
      1oz/30g soda bread crumbs
      1 tsp sage
      1oz/30g oatmeal
      Salt and black pepper
      1 egg

Soak lentils overnight in enough water to cover. Cook in same water until soft and water is absorbed. Beat until smooth.

Heat butter and fry onions, skinned tomatoes, and apple until soft. Add to the lentils, with soda bread crumbs, oatmeal, sage and seasoning.

Bind with egg and press into a greased loaf tin. Cover with greased paper.

Bake in the centre of an oven, 400F, 200C Gas Mark 6 for 45-60 minutes.

LENTIL CUTLETS   Serves 4

Ingredients:

      8oz/225g lentils
      2oz/50g butter
      2 chopped onions
      2 large tomatoes, skinned
      1 small peeled, cored and chopped apple
      1oz/30g soda bread crumbs
      1 tsp sage
      1oz/30g oatmeal
      Salt and black pepper
      1 egg

To coat:

      2oz/50g soda bread crumbs
      A little beaten egg

Soak lentils overnight in enough water to cover. Cook in same water until soft and water is absorbed. Beat until smooth.

Heat butter and fry onions, skinned tomatoes, and apple until quite soft. Add to the lentils, together with the breadcrumbs, sage, oatmeal and seasoning.

Bind with the egg and form into cutlet shapes.
Roll in breadcrumbs after brushing with beaten egg and fry or bake in oven,
425F, 220C, Gas Mark 7 until crisp and brown.

RICE & PARSLEY CHEESE   Serves 2

Ingredients:
>   2 tblsp oil
>   1 onion, chopped
>   1 clove garlic
>   1 cup brown rice
>   ½tsp basil or marjoram
>   3 tblsp finely chopped parsley
>   Good pinch of turmeric
>   2 cups hot water
>   ½cup cheese, grated

Heat the oil and sauté the onion and chopped garlic. Add rice and cook for 3
minutes, stirring constantly. (Grains should all be golden).
Add basil, turmeric and parsley to hot water and pour 1 cup on to rice.
Cover and allow to simmer for a few minutes. Add remaining cup of water and
simmer gradually until it is all absorbed about 30-40 minutes.
Just before rice has finished cooking add half the cheese. When melted remove
from heat, add rest of cheese and serve.

EGG PILAU   Serves 2

Ingredients:
>   1 onion, chopped
>   1 clove garlic, chopped
>   4 tblsp olive oil
>   1 cup brown rice, uncooked
>   2-3 cups hot water
>   ½ tsp allspice powder
>   3 cloves
>   ½ tsp cinnamon powder
>   1 tsp salt
>   2 eggs, hard boiled

Sauté onion and garlic in olive oil. Add rice and cook until transparent, stirring
constantly.

Pour hot water over spices and salt and add ½ cup of this mix to the pan of rice. Cover and simmer gently for 10 minutes. Gradually add remaining liquid till all is absorbed and rice is tender, (about 20-25 minutes). Serve hot, garnished with chopped egg.

LENTIL PANCAKES   Serves 2

Ingredients:

    10fl.oz/275ml water
    4oz/100g lentils
    1 onion chopped
    1 tomato, pulped
    3 tblsp oil
    ½tsp. salt
    Pinch of thyme
    3 tblsp ground rice
    1 egg, beaten

Wash and cover lentils with water. Leave overnight.
Add onion, tomato, 1 tablespoon oil and seasoning. Cover pan and simmer gently for 2 hours.
Stir in 2 tablespoons ground rice and keep stirring for 10 minutes until mixture is stiff. Allow to cool.
Form into flat cakes. Dip in beaten egg, roll in remaining ground rice and sauté in remaining oil till brown on both sides.

INDIAN SAVOURY   Serves 1

Ingredients:

    1-2oz/25-50g brown rice
    ½tblsp olive oil
    1 diced onion
    1 crushed clove garlic
    1/3 tsp ground coriander
    1/3 tsp ground cumin
    2 finely diced green chillies
    ½ green pepper, de-seeded and sliced
    2oz/50g okra
    5oz/150g cooked chickpeas
    10fl.oz/275ml vegetable stock
    Fresh parsley to garnish

Wash rice well in plenty of cold water. Drain.

Sauté rice in olive oil with onion, garlic, spices, chillies, green pepper and thinly sliced okra. Stir well for 10 minutes.

Stir in the cooked chickpeas, add stock, cover and simmer for 10 minutes.

Remove any scum that has formed on the top of the pan, cover and simmer for another 20 minutes. Serve, garnished with sprigs of fresh parsley.

LAMB & JUNIPER PIE   Serves 6

Ingredients:

    2 tblsps olive oil
    2lb/900g lamb fillet, cubed
    1 onion, peeled and chopped
    1 clove garlic, crushed
    14oz/400g can tomatoes
    14oz/400g can red kidney beans, drained and washed
    ½tsp cinnamon
    ½tsp juniper berries, crushed
    Salt and pepper to taste

Oat Pastry:

    8oz/225g wholemeal flour
    1oz/30g rolled oats
    Pinch of salt
    4oz/100g butter
    Beaten egg to glaze

Heat oil in a saucepan, fry lamb cubes until browned. Remove lamb from pan. Add onion and garlic to the pan and fry for 3 minutes. Return lamb to pan, add tomatoes, kidney beans, cinnamon, juniper berries and seasoning.

Bring to boil, reduce heat, cover and cook gently for 40 minutes until lamb is tender. Spoon into a 2 pint/1 litre pie dish and leave to cool.

Place flour, oats and a pinch of salt into a bowl. Rub in butter. Stir in 4 tablespoons water and mix to a soft dough. Knead lightly on a floured surface and roll out until a little larger than the pie dish to form pie lid.

Roll out a strip of pastry about 1"/2.5cm wide, brush edge of dish with water and place strip on edge of dish. Brush top of strip with water. Place pie lid on top of dish, press edges together well, trim pastry. Knock up and flute edge. Cook at 400F, 200C, Gas Mark 6 for 55 minutes.

CURRIED LAMB & LENTILS   Serves 6

Ingredients:

> 2lb/900g lean lamb cut from leg or shoulder
> 4 tblsp olive oil
> 2 onions peeled and thinly sliced
> 2 cloves garlic, peeled and crushed
> 1 tsp ground cumin
> 1 tsp turmeric
> 1 tsp chilli powder
> 2 tsp ground coriander
> 1 tsp ground ginger
> ½tsp ground cinnamon
> 20fl.oz/550ml water
> 7oz/200g can plum tomatoes
> 8oz/225g lentils
> 5fl.oz/150ml natural yoghurt

Trim any fat from the meat and cut into 1"/2.5cm cubes.

Heat the oil and fry the meat in small batches for 2-3 minutes to seal. Remove with a draining spoon before adding the next batch.

When all meat has been fried and set aside, add onions to the pan, adding more oil if necessary, and cook over gentle heat until soft, stirring occasionally.

Add garlic and spices and cook for a further minute.

Return meat to the pan and pour in water and tomatoes with their juice. Stir in lentils and season.

Bring slowly to boil, lower heat, cover pan and simmer for 90 minutes until lentils are tender. Serve topped with yoghurt.

YOGHURT LAMB KEBABS   Serves 4

Ingredients:

      6fl.oz/175ml natural yoghurt
      1 tblsp olive oil
      Juice of 2 lemons
      1 tsp salt
      2 cloves garlic, crushed
      1 tsp salt
      ½tsp ground black pepper
      ½tsp ground ginger
      ½tsp ground cumin
      ½tsp turmeric
      24oz/700g lamb, cut in 1"/2.5cm cubes
      1 large onion cut in quarters and divided in leaves.

Put all ingredients except lamb and onion in a bowl and stir well until mixed. Add meat and onion and stir until evenly coated in the marinade. Cover and refrigerate for 4-6 hours.

Drain meat off and thread, with onions, onto skewers. Cook over glowing charcoal or under a hot grill until meat is brown and tender. Baste with marinade and turn during cooking. Slide kebabs off skewers directly on to serving plates.

LENTIL COTTAGE PIE   Serves 1

Ingredients:

      2oz/50g whole brown lentils
      1 onion, diced
      1 carrot, diced
      6 Brussels sprouts
      1 medium parsnip, diced
      10fl.oz/275ml vegetable stock
      1 large potato

Boil lentils in plenty of water for 25 minutes.

Place diced onion, carrot, parsnips and sprouts in a sauce pan with a little stock, and cook in their own steam over a moderate heat for 15 minutes.

Chop potato and boil until cooked.

Use olive oil to lightly cover an ovenproof dish.

Drain lentils, mix with vegetables and place in the dish with the remaining stock and parsley.

Cook in a pre heated oven at 350F, 180C, Gas Mark 4 for 10 minutes.

Mash the potato, adding salt and pepper to taste. Cover the vegetables with mashed potatoes, return to oven for a further 20 minutes.

EGGS FLORENTINE   Serves 4

Ingredients:

        Microwave on full power throughout.

        2 medium potatoes, scrubbed

        7oz/200g frozen spinach

        1oz/30g butter

        ½tsp nutmeg, grated

        2 eggs, size 4

        Paprika

Prick the potatoes all over. Put on a plate and cook for 15 minutes or until tender.

Put spinach in a bowl, covered with pierced cling film. Cook for 10 minutes stirring once, until thawed. Transfer to a sieve and squeeze out water with a spoon.

Slice the top off each potato. Carefully scoop out the flesh with a spoon, leaving a shell of potato about ½ inch/1.25cm thick inside the skin. Add potato to spinach and mix in the butter, nutmeg and paprika to taste.

Spoon mixture back into potato skins, leaving a centre hollow. Break 1 egg into each hollow. Pierce yolk carefully with a cocktail stick. Put potatoes on a plate and cook for 1-2 minutes, or until egg white is just set. Sprinkle with paprika and garnish.

STUFFED CABBAGE ROLLS   Serves 4

Ingredients:

8oz/225g green lentils
12 large green cabbage leaves
1 tblsp olive oil
2 medium onions, sliced
2 tblsp tomato purée
1 large red pepper, cored, de-seeded and chopped finely
1 tsp ground mixed spice
Salt and pepper to taste
10fl.oz/275ml vegetable stock
14oz/450g can tomatoes and juice

Put lentils in a saucepan, cover with cold water, and bring to boil and simmer for 20-25 minutes until tender.

Meanwhile, cut out thick 'woody' veins at base of each cabbage leaf by cutting a 'V' shape. Blanch leaves in boiling water for 4-5 minutes. Drain and set aside to cool. Heat oil in a saucepan, add onions and cook gently for 5 minutes until soft. Add tomato purée, red pepper, mixed spice, salt and pepper. Cook for 2-3 minutes.

Drain lentils, add to onion mix and stir well. Remove from heat. Divide mix evenly between each cabbage leaf and roll up to form a parcel. Pack stuffed cabbage leaves closely together in a greased baking dish.

Mix together vegetable stock, tinned tomatoes and juice. Pour over cabbage rolls. Cover and bake at 350F, 180C, Gas Mark 4 for 40 minutes. Serve hot.

POTATO SALAD WITH CHIVES   Serves 4

Ingredients:

1 tblsp olive oil
1 clove garlic, crushed
½tsp turmeric
1lb/450g diced boiled potatoes
1 tblsp fresh chives, chopped
4 tblsp home made mayonnaise

Heat oil in a pan. Gently fry the garlic clove for several minutes Blend in turmeric then remove from heat.

Cool slightly then pour over the potatoes, coating each piece. Mix in chives and mayonnaise. Serve chilled.

MIXED UP SALAD   Serves 4

Ingredients:

>   8oz/225g beansprouts
>   4oz/100g water chestnuts
>   4oz/100g pineapple, fresh or tinned, drained
>   ¼tsp ground cumin
>   ¼tsp ground coriander
>   3 tblsp mayonnaise
>   Pinch ground coriander to garnish

Combine beansprouts, water chestnuts and pineapple and mix well.
Stir cumin, and ground coriander into mayonnaise and pour the mixture over
the salad.
Toss well, garnish with a pinch of ground coriander and serve at once.

MILLET DROPS

Ingredients:

>   ½ cup millet
>   Water to cover
>   1 egg white
>   Pinch of salt

Soak millet overnight in water. Drain off liquid and set aside.
Whip egg white with 1 tablespoon of liquid set aside. Add pinch of salt and
stir in millet to make a thin batter.
Drop one teaspoon on a heated lightly oiled pan or a hot dry griddle. Brown
well on both sides.
Serve lightly buttered.

PIQUANT SPREAD

Ingredients:

½ cup cottage cheese
¼cup goats milk
2 tsp grated raw onion
Paprika, salt or celery seeds to taste

Soak cheese in fresh milk, add onion then blend in liquidiser or beat thoroughly with eggbeater.
Add paprika, salt or celery seeds to taste. Press into screw top jar and chill. Use as a spread on rice cakes, soda bread etc.

SHRIMP SPREAD

Ingredients:

20 fresh shrimps
1 tblsp butter
Sprinkle of paprika
Grating of nutmeg
1 tsp melted butter

Skin and chop shrimps, pound in a mortar or bowl.
Beat together butter and paprika and a grating of nutmeg. Add shrimps and mix well. Press into small glass dish or jar and cover with 1 teaspoon melted butter and prepared greaseproof paper. Put weight on top and chill for 24 hours.

STAGE 4 DIET & RECIPES

At last! This is the final phase of your fight against Candida. Look back at the questionnaires to remind yourself of the problems you had when you started and you will be surprised at just how many things you have forgotten.

Remember that having Candida is a bit like being an alcoholic – you are never cured, you will always have to be careful. However, if you treat your body and diet with respect you should remain well on this regime. If you do slip back into your old eating habits you will probably find all of your symptoms returning.

Now incorporate the following foods into your existing diet, one item a day as before. Remember to always rotate your food as much as possible, within your diet.

VEGETABLES   Beetroot, Sweetcorn, Yam (sweet potato)

FISH   Cod, Turbot, Whiting

FRUIT   Blackcurrants, Date, Fig, Grapefruit, Loganberry, Nectarine, Orange, Raspberry, Redcurrants, Pear, Quince, Raisin

GRAINS   Bulgar Wheat, Cornmeal, Wheat, Wheatgerm

NUTS   Brazil, Pistachio, Walnut

MISCELLANEOUS
                Citric Acid (as a preservative) Coconut Milk, Corn Oil,
                Corn Starch, Soy Sauce

HOT & SOUR SOUP   Serves 6

Ingredients:
    60fl.oz/1.75 litres chicken stock or water
    1 green chilli, sliced
    4 strips lemon peel
    Juice from 1 lemon.
    4 slices fresh ginger
    4 cloves garlic
    Vegetable, garnish
    4 spring onions, trimmed and sliced
    1 small carrot cut in matchsticks
    4 oz./100g fresh beansprouts
    2 tblsp fresh coriander, chopped

Put chicken stock or water in a large pan with the chilli, strips of lemon, ginger
and garlic. Cover and simmer for 15 minutes.
Strain, then return stock to the pan with the lemon juice.
Just before serving, return to the boil then stir in the vegetable garnish and
coriander. Simmer for 1–2 minutes then serve immediately.

NOTE:
Before serving, liquidise the mixture to make it thicker, if preferred.

SPINACH SOUP   Serves 4

Ingredients:

      1lb/450g spinach
      20fl.oz/550ml water
      1 large potato
      1 small onion
      20fl.oz/550ml soy milk
      Pinch of salt
      Grated nutmeg

Wash spinach thoroughly in several changes of water to remove any grit. Put in a large pan with the water.

Scrub and dice the potato, finely chop the onion and add to the spinach. Simmer until potato is tender. Remove and cool.

Liquidise or rub through sieve.

Return to pan, add milk, salt and grating of nutmeg. Reheat without boiling, and serve.

TOMATO SOUP   Serves 4

Ingredients:

      1 small onion
      1 tblsp oil
      1lb/450g tomatoes
      1 medium potato
      Pinch of basil
      20fl.oz/550ml stock or water
      15fl.oz/425ml soy milk
      Salt to taste

Peel and chop onion. Heat oil in pan and sauté onion.

Cut up tomatoes and potatoes and add to onions. Sprinkle with basil.

Pour on stock or water and simmer for about 15 minutes until potato is tender.

Cool and liquidise and strain or rub through sieve.

Return to pan, add milk and salt to taste and reheat without boiling.

QUICK VEGETABLE SOUP   Serves 3

Ingredients:

     2 tblsp oil
     1lb/450g carrots
     1 turnip
     1 small parsnip
     2 medium onions
     20fl.oz/550ml stock or water
     1 sprig each marjoram, thyme, and half a bay leaf
     10fl.oz/275ml soy milk
     1 tblsp parsley

Heat oil in pan and grate in the carrots, turnips, parsley and onions. Sauté together lightly.
Add stock and herbs tied in muslin. Simmer gently for a few minutes until tender.
Remove herbs, add milk, salt to taste and reheat.
Add finely chopped parsley just before serving.

ITALIAN COD   Serves 1

Ingredients:

     4oz/100g frozen cod steak
     8oz/225g canned tomatoes
     1oz/30g chopped onion
     1 tblsp bran
     1oz/30g chopped green pepper
     Salt and pepper
     Pinch dried oregano or ½ tsp chopped fresh oregano

Place frozen cod steak in small ovenproof dish or casserole.
Chop canned tomatoes and mix with tomato juice, onion, bran, green pepper and seasoning to taste.
Spoon over fish and bake in a moderate oven for 30 minutes. Serve with a jacket potato.

FISH ON A DISH   Serves 1

Ingredients:
>   Microwave on high power throughout
>   1 small carrot
>   1 small courgette
>   1 small turnip
>   1 egg yolk
>   2 tsp lemon juice
>   1oz/30g butter
>   6oz/175g cod cutlet
>   Sprig of parsley

Coarsely grate prepared carrot, courgette and turnip.
Mix the egg yolk and lemon juice in a small bowl with a little seasoning.
Cut butter into pieces and melt in another small bowl for about 30 seconds.
Gradually pour the melted butter onto the egg yolk and lemon juice mixture in a thin steady stream, whisking continuously.
Cook for 30 seconds until thick, stir well and reserve.
Place the cutlet on a microproof serving plate, cover with cling film, pierce and cook for another 90 seconds.
Peel back wrapping and spoon grated vegetables all around the fish. Re-cover and cook for 90 seconds or until fish flakes when it's pressed with a knife.
Reheat sauce for 20 seconds and serve with fish and vegetables. Garnish with parsley and serve.

DILL & ORANGE TROUT   Serves 3

Ingredients:
>   3 trout fillets
>   Salt and black pepper
>   Rind and juice of 1 orange
>   2 tsp fresh dill
>   Few chives, chopped
>   A little butter

Lay trout fillets in greased oven dish, and season lightly with salt and black pepper. Cover with rind and juice of orange and sprinkle with dill and chives. Top each fillet with a knob of butter and bake uncovered for 7-10 minutess in a hot oven.
Garnish with orange slices.

TRAWLERMAN'S SUPPER

Serves 4

Ingredients:

      4oz/100g thinly sliced onion
      2oz/50g sliced leek
      2 tsp butter
      14oz/400g tin tomatoes
      1 tblsp. tomato purée
      1oz/30g wholemeal flour
      ½tsp. dried marjoram
      Good pinch dried sage
      1lb/450g cooked, sliced, unpeeled potatoes
      1lb/450g skinned cod fillets
      1oz/30g toasted soda bread crumbs
      Good pinch dried marjoram
      ¼tsp black pepper
      ¼tsp salt

Preheat oven to 350F, 180C, Gas Mark 4.

In a pan, Sauté thinly sliced onion and sliced leek in butter until soft. Stir in tin tomatoes, tomato purée, wholemeal flour, marjoram and sage. Cook for 2-3 minutes.

Transfer to a shallow ovenproof dish and cover with potatoes. Arrange cod fillets on top. Sprinkle with soda bread crumbs, pinch of dried marjoram, ground black pepper and salt.

Cover and bake for 30 minutes.

SALMON PATTIES

Serves 4

Ingredients:

      1lb/450g tin of salmon, red or pink
      2oz/50g wheatgerm
      2-3oz/50-75g whole wheat flour
      2 eggs, beaten
      2oz/50g stone ground corn meal
      4oz/100g onion, chopped
      2oz/50g pepper, chopped
      1 tblsp lemon juice

Carefully remove large bones from fish and flake well.
Mix all ingredients together and form into 8 patties.
Brown in a little olive oil on medium heat for 15 minutes

COD LAYER PIE   Serves 4

Ingredients:

> 1lb/450g fresh cod fillets
> 2 tblsp parsley, finely chopped
> 4oz/100g onion, chopped
> 2lb/900g potatoes
> 2 tblsp butter
> ½ cup water

Wash fish and cut into 2"/5cm pieces. Lay in an oiled pie dish, sprinkle with
a layer of chopped parsley, then a layer of chopped onion. Carry on with layers
of fish, parsley and onion until they have all been used.
Steam potatoes, rub through a sieve, beat in a little butter and mix with the
water to make a soft paste.
Cover fish layers with potato, dot with remaining butter and bake at 375F,
190C, Gas Mark 5 for about 20 minutes until lightly browned.

ORANGE & CORIANDER RICE   Serves 4

Ingredients:

> 6oz/175g long grain brown rice
> 7 fl.oz/200ml orange juice
> 10 fl.oz/275ml chicken stock
> 2 tsp coriander seeds, crushed★
> Pinch of powdered saffron or turmeric#
> Pinch of salt

Rinse rice under cold running water until the water runs clear. This removes
the excess starch and prevents the rice turning sticky.
Place the orange juice and chicken stock in a large pan and bring to the boil.
Stir in the rice, crushed coriander and saffron or turmeric. Season with salt,
return to the boil, then reduce the heat to a steady simmer.
Cover the pan and cook until all the liquid has been absorbed (about 15
minutes).

★ Make sure you use crushed coriander seeds, not ground coriander. To crush the coriander seeds, either use a pestle and mortar or the end of a rolling pin in a bowl.

\# Saffron gives the dish a subtle flavour and delightful colour. Turmeric is a cheaper substitute, gives a tronger, spicy flavour and a darker colour.

SPICED BEAN POT   Serves 4

Ingredients:

> 4oz/100g peeled, chopped onions
> 2 tsp olive oil
> 1–2 tsp mild chilli powder
> 14oz/400g tin tomatoes with juice
> 1 tblsp tomato puree
> 2oz/50g wholemeal flour
> 10fl.oz/275ml water
> ½tsp garlic granules
> ¼tsp salt
> 8oz/225g courgettes, sliced
> 6oz/175g red peppers, sliced
> 6oz/175g green peppers, sliced
> 15oz/425g tin red kidney beans, drained and rinsed
> 15oz/425g tin haricot beans, drained and rinsed
> 8oz/225g sweetcorn kernels

Heat oil in a large pan and stir in onions. Cook until soft. Stir in chilli powder and cook for 1 minute.

Add tin tomatoes with juice, tomato purée and wholemeal flour. Mix well. Blend in water, garlic granules, salt, courgettes, red and green peppers.

Add rinsed and drained kidney beans, haricot beans and sweetcorn. Bring to the boil, cover and simmer for 10–12 minutes until vegetables are tender. Serve, sprinkled with black pepper. (This dish can be frozen for up to 12 months.)

WHOLEMEAL VEGETABLE PIE   Serves 4

Ingredients:

> 8oz/225g wholemeal flour
> ½ tsp. salt
> 4oz/100g butter
> 4 tblsp cold water

FILLING:

>   2 tblsp olive oil
>   1 large onion, chopped
>   3 medium carrots, finely chopped
>   10oz/275g courgettes, finely chopped
>   15oz/425g can tomatoes
>   Salt and pepper

Heat the oil in a saucepan, add onions and carrot, then stir, cover and fry gently for 10 minutes.

Add courgettes and tomatoes. Stir well, cover and cook for a further 10-15 minutes until tender. Season with salt and pepper.

Put the mixture in a 2 pint/1 litre pie dish and leave to cool. Preheat oven to 400F, 200C, Gas Mark 6.

Mix flour and salt in a bowl. Cut butter into small pieces and rub in with fingertips until mixture resembles breadcrumbs. Add water and press mixture together to make a dough.

Roll pastry out quite thickly into the same shape as the pie dish but 1"/2.5cm larger all round. Cut off this 1"/2.5cm strip, dampen the rim of the pie dish and place the pastry strip on top.

Dampen pastry strip then put large piece of pastry on top, pressing edges down firmly to seal. Make a couple of holes in the pastry for the steam to escape, and bake for 25-30 minutes or until golden brown.

TOMATO FLOWER FRITTER   Serves 4

Ingredients:

>   4 tomatoes
>   1 small cauliflower
>   4oz/100g wholemeal flour
>   Good pinch of salt
>   1 egg
>   Vegetable oil for frying
>   Cayenne pepper

Rub tomatoes through sieve and if necessary, add a little water to make 5fl.oz/150ml.

Divide the cauliflower into neat sprigs — try to keep them uniform in size. Cook in boiling salted water until just soft, but unbroken. Drain well.

Sieve the flour and salt together. Add the well-beaten egg and gradually beat in the tomato purée.

Put the pieces of cauliflower into this batter and, when well coated, drop in boiling vegetable oil and cook until crisp and brown. Dust with cayenne pepper and serve at once.

STUFFED GREEN PEPPERS   Serves 4

Ingredients:

> 4 small green peppers
> 6oz/175g frozen smoked haddock fillets
> 4oz/100g long grain brown rice
> 4oz/100g sweetcorn
> ¼ tsp dried thyme
> Salt and black pepper
> 5fl.oz/150ml yoghurt

Cut tops off peppers and remove seeds.
Blanch peppers in lightly salted boiling water for 5 minutes. Drain and arrange in an ovenproof dish.
Cook fish fillets, following directions on packet. Remove any skin or bones and flake fish.
Mix fish with rice, sweetcorn, thyme, seasoning and yoghurt. Spoon mixture into peppers and cook in a moderately hot oven, 375F, 190C, Gas Mark 5 for 30 minutes. Serve hot.

WHEAT BISCUITS   Makes 12

Ingredients:

> 1lb/450g whole wheat flour
> 4 tsp baking powder
> 3fl.oz/75ml unrefined vegetable oil
> ½ tsp salt
> 6-8fl.oz/175-225ml water

Mix together all dry ingredients. Add oil and mix well (very important).
Add enough water to make dough that is soft but not sticky and mix just enough to moisten the dry ingredients.
Using hands only, pat dough out to ¾ inch/2cm thick on a floured board. Using a biscuit cutter cut out 12 biscuit shapes and place on a lightly oiled baking sheet.
Bake for 20 minutes or until done at 450F, 230C, Gas Mark 8.

ADDITIONAL ADVICE

Allergies are often caused by a calcium deficiency so make sure you eat plenty of calcium rich foods within the confines of your diet. Good food sources of calcium for Candida patients are: live yoghurt, dark green leafy vegetables, broccoli, citrus fruits, canned fish with edible bones, dried peas and beans. When allergies are very troublesome, the remedy Urticalcin can be very useful. This will complement any other remedies in your current programme.

Remember that 'milk makes mucous' and be always wary of any dairy produce as this could well increase **catarrh**. Avoid salt, wheat and milk. Eat lots of common watercress. Another helpful idea is to put a cut onion in a dish on the bedside table overnight. You will inhale the fumes while you are sleeping which should greatly reduce the severity of 'morning catarrh'. Swiss Garlic Capsules can also be very useful and will work with any other remedies you are taking.

To help increase your immunity to **colds** and **flu**, eat plenty of salads with watercress, horseradish, gardencress and nasturtiums. Swiss Garlic Capsules can also help to improve your resistance.

Cheese, eggs and potatoes can increase **constipation** so it is best to avoid these until the problem is under control. Also, make sure you drink plenty of water to help soften the motion. Exercise, such as brisk walking, is very helpful if you can manage it.

Avoiding citrus fruit should help **cystitis** and drinking cranberry juice is particularly beneficial.

Reduce your tea and coffee intake to help relieve **depression** and **mouth ulcers**.

Many **eczema** patients are allergic to eggs, dairy produce, salt and wheat. It would be a good idea to leave these out of your diet for at least a month. Use this as a trial period to see if there is an improvement in your condition. You should not consider omitting anything from your diet for less than a month, to give it a really fair trial. Skin conditions often require longer than most other problems before they show an improvement, so don't expect to see any change overnight.

A high protein diet can often help people with **eye problems**. A three-ounce portion of cooked fish or poultry can deliver between fifteen and twenty five grams of protein. Most seeds, such as pumpkin, sunflower and sesame, contain a good amount of protein but seeds do not have as much fat content as nuts, which is another high protein food.

Recurring **headaches** can suggest low blood sugar or high blood pressure. Have you had these checked recently? Slow, deep breathing while sipping a cup of peppermint tea can often relieve headaches. Alternatively you can apply a warm, not hot, shower to the nape of the neck and upper spine. Do not forget to have your eyes tested to ensure that your headaches are not being caused by eyestrain.

A strict anti Candida diet is essential for the treatment of **oral thrush** and frequent gargling with diluted Molkosan will help to fight the infection.

Leaving tea, coffee, and chocolate out of your diet should help relieve **PMT** and **breast tenderness**. Try using a coffee substitute such as Bambu.

Most symptoms are aggravated by stress, and **psoriasis** is probably worse than any other. Try joining yoga or relaxation classes to help bring your problems under control.

If you have trouble **sleeping** at night, avoid eating for at least two hours before going to bed. Omit coffee, tea and chocolate from your diet. Just before retiring, apply a cold water pack, or cold flannel to the back of the head and neck. Remember that an hour's sleep before midnight is worth two hours sleep afterwards.

If you suffer from frequent **sore throats**, don't overlook the old fashioned remedy of gargling with salt water – it really helps.

When **vaginal thrush** is a nuisance, before going to bed insert two teaspoonfuls of natural live yoghurt into the vagina, with the aid of a tampon. Put a little witch hazel or concentrated whey, such as Molkosan, onto a clean sanitary towel and place over the vagina. It will help to relieve the terrible itching. Avoid bath oils, shower gels, foam baths, soap and talc in the vaginal area. Always use white toilet paper as the dyes used in coloured paper can cause irritation. Only wear underwear made from natural fibres. Avoid tights, leggings, trousers or tight jeans, as they can cause excessive sweating and will increase the problem.

If **wind** is a problem, (in either direction!) you can help matters by avoiding fried food and try not to eat fruit and vegetables at the same meal. Also, beware of some types of pulse or fibre.

Try to improve your **memory** by reducing your consumption of meat, eggs and cheese; instead eat more vegetables and salads. Use less common salt, but always try to substitute it with herbs including Herbamare and Trocomare.

CONVERSION TABLE

Based on a conversion factor of
1 oz. = 28.35g

Based on a conversion factor of
1 fl.oz = 28.41ml

1 oz	–	30g	5 fl.oz	–	150ml
2 oz	–	50g	8 fl.oz	–	225ml
3 oz	–	75g	10 fl.oz	–	275ml
4 oz	–	100g	15 fl.oz	–	425ml
5 oz	–	150g	20 fl.oz	–	550ml
6 oz	–	175g	25 fl.oz	–	700ml
7 oz	–	200g	30 fl.oz	–	850ml
8 oz	–	225g	35 fl.oz	–	1 litre
9 oz	–	250g	60 fl.oz	–	1.75 litres
10 oz	–	275g			
11 oz	–	300g			
12 oz	–	350g			
13 oz	–	375g			
14 oz	–	400g			
15 oz	–	425g			
16 oz	–	450g			

RECOMMENDED PRODUCTS

If you are unable to find the recommended products locally, contact Bioforce for your nearest stockist:

BIOFORCE (UK) Ltd
2 Brewster Place
Irvine
Ayrshire KA11 5DD
Telephone: 01294 277344
Fax: 01294 277922